Psychiatric Disorders with a Biochemical Basis

Psychiatric Disorders with a Biochemical Basis

including pharmacology, toxicology and nutritional aspects

David Donaldson, MB, ChB, MRCP, FRCPath

Consultant in Chemical Pathology
East Surrey Hospital, Redhill, Surrey
and Crawley Hospital, Crawley,
West Sussex, UK

The Parthenon Publishing Group
International Publishers in Medicine, Science & Technology

NEW YORK · LONDON

Published in the USA by
The Parthenon Publishing Group Inc.
One Blue Hill Plaza
PO Box 1564, Pearl River
New York 10965, USA

Published in the UK by
The Parthenon Publishing Group Limited
Casterton Hall, Carnforth
Lancs. LA6 2LA, UK

First published 1998

Library of Congress Cataloging-in-Publication Data
Donaldson, David.
        Psychiatric disorders with a biochemical basis : including pharmacology,
toxicology and nutritional aspects / David Donaldson.
             p.   cm.
        Includes bibliographical references and index.
        ISBN 1-85070-789-8 (hardcover)
        1. Mental illness—Pathophysiology. 2. Behavioral toxicology.
        3. Psychological manifestations of general diseases. 4. Central Nervous
System—drug effects. 5. Biological Psychiatry.
        [DNLM: 1. Mental Disorders—chemically induced. 2. Mental
Disorders—physiopathology.]
        RC455.4.B5D66   1997
        616.89′07—dc21
        DNLM/DLC
        for Library of Congress   97-7656
                                                                                                    CIP

British Library Cataloguing in Publication Data
Donaldson, David
        Psychiatric disorders with a biochemical basis : including pharmacology,
        toxicology and nutritional aspects
        1. Psychiatry 2. Clinical biochemistry
        I. Title
        616.8′9
        ISBN 1-85070-789-8

Typeset by Martin Lister Publishing Services, Carnforth, UK
Printed and bound by Bookcraft (Bath) Ltd., Midsomer Norton, UK

Contents

Foreword

The association of mental disorders with physical disease has always attracted the interest of psychiatrists, but the degree of their actual involvement in this field has waxed and waned over the years. Although earlier in the century Kraepelin, together with many other major contributors to psychiatric knowledge, believed that physical illnesses frequently showed characteristic mental symptoms, these came to be considered as being within the realm of general medicine rather than of psychiatry. However, the more recent emergence of liaison psychiatry as a subspecialty has been a tangible recognition of the common ground where collaboration between general physicians and psychiatrists is essential in the diagnosis and management of such presentations.

This book gives an overview of psychiatric disorders with a biochemical basis and biological disorders with a psychiatric component. It examines metabolic, biochemical and endocrine disturbances, including sections on pharmacological, toxicological and nutritional aspects – as well as the laboratory investigations of psychiatric disorders. It is written in a clear, concise, readable style and the text is illuminated by illustrative case studies, drawing throughout on the most up-to-date research literature. It will not only assist general physicians and psychiatrists in their day-to-day practice but also will be a valuable source of information to both undergraduate and post-graduate students.

The author combines a wide range of clinical experience with a particular interest in psychiatry and an enthusiasm for teaching. His scientific expertise in chemical pathology brings an important new dimension to the study of this field.

Mounir Ekdawi
MB, ChB, DPM, FRCPsych
August 1997

Preface

The brain is structurally and functionally immensely complex – but is, nevertheless, gradually yielding the secrets of its physics and chemistry. Exactly as J.W.L. Thudichum ('father of neurochemistry') predicted in 1884, it has been by way of continued application of our growing knowledge of brain biochemistry to the common psychiatric disorders, to which the human race is subject, that we are slowly and steadily gaining clearer, deeper and more detailed understanding of actual mechanisms involved in the disease processes. It is, in general, these disorders that have been discussed in books on the biochemical basis of psychiatry. However, the theme and contents of the present volume are somewhat different. The author became interested in the association between often relatively small changes in those biochemical indices routinely available from any clinical chemistry laboratory and the aberrations of mood (and the sometimes minor changes in other aspects of psychological function) which are revealed only after very carefully listening to the patient's 'story'. Analysis of such observations, taken in conjunction with detailed clinical observation, permit important and interesting clinical conclusions; it is, indeed, almost too easy to gloss over some of the subtle changes of mind, without realising their true clinical significance. The initial interest grew and there followed a publication on the laboratory tests available on blood and urine which were not only of value in establishing or confirming a clinical diagnosis but also for assessing progress in response to appropriate medication or other therapy. The interest yet further developed as more case histories accumulated; the material then came to form the basis of a chapter in a textbook of clinical biochemistry. The chapter, as originally written, was much too long for its immediate purpose – and yet the unused material was of too great an interest to ignore. Encouragement from friends and colleagues in relevant specialities resulted in an update and expansion of the original material with the addition of further chapters to produce the present volume.

The clinical section of the book is an exposition on 'secondary psychiatry, defined as comprising the psychological and psychiatric consequences of sometimes minor changes in inorganic or organic constituents of the body (caused by biochemical, pharmacological, toxicological, or nutritional disturbances) and which may be detected at an early stage of disease by examining blood and/or urine. Not discussed in detail in this volume, however, are the psychological/psychiatric sequelae of microbiological infections nor the mental consequences of physically based disorders such as head injury and space occupying intracranial lesions.

Throughout the evolutionary process of my interest in this topic I have received help and encouragement from a number of people. Special thanks go to Dr David Williams (Consultant Chemical Patholo-gist, Royal Berkshire Hospital, Reading, Berkshire) and Professor Vincent Marks (Dean of Medicine and Emeritus Professor of Clinical Biochemistry, University of Surrey, Guildford, Surrey) for initially stimulating be to crystallise my thoughts and ideas into a tangible presentation. I would particularly like to thank my colleague and friend Professor John Dickerson (Emeritus Professor of Human Nutri-tion, University of Surrey, Guildford, Surrey) for his help and encour-agement throughout the preparation of this book and especially for his suggestions and collaboration in writing the chapter on 'Psychiatric consequences of disorders of the developing brain'. I would also like to thank my long-standing colleague Dr Mounir Ekdawi (formerly Consultant Psychiatrist, East Surrey Hospital, Redhill, Surrey) for his enthusiasm in acting as catalyst in encouraging and furthering my interest in psychiatry over many years and also for generously writing a Foreword. I express grateful thanks to other medical colleagues - not only for their willing co-operation in allowing me to study in detail some of their patients, but also for giving me their kind permission to publish some of the case histories herein. Consultant colleagues at East Surrey Hospital, Redhill, Surrey and some at Crawley Hospital, Crawley, West Sussex who have helped in this way include: Dr Richard Bailey, Mr John Hale, Dr Tony Hicklin, Dr Paul Jenkins and Dr Eileen Phillips. In addition, it is a pleasure to acknowledge the particu-lar contribution of Dr Julia Peters. Last, but not least, my thanks go to Dr Helen Lee of the Parthenon Publishing Group Limited for most valuable, thoughtful, constructive discussion and also for her consider-able patience and expertise in translating my own documentations into a professional product.

David Donaldson
MB, ChB, MRCP, FRCPath
August 1997

1
Introduction

Every illness, whether basically psychiatric or biological, possesses an emotional aspect as at least part of its clinical presentation. The latter could, however, comprise the major component of the disorder where there is essentially a psycho-social, family or personality problem; in particular, the illness might be reactive to certain events or to a situation. On the other hand, the emotional aspect could be a reaction to any illness, which might itself be predominantly biological (e.g. depression and/or anxiety following a myocardial infarction). Although another possibility is that there might be close and integral involvement between the mental state and basic biological processes (e.g. depression or confusion as an accompaniment of the hypercalcaemia of primary hyperparathyroidism). In yet other instances the mental features could be secondary to a microbiological infection (e.g. lethargy as the one and only complaint of a patient with an 'almost subclinical' episode of viral hepatitis) or could be attributed to the side-effects of a pharmacological agent, being either prescribed as therapy (e.g. memory impairment and confusion following bedtime dosage with the short-acting benzodiazepine, triazolam) or taken for some other reason (e.g. decreased alertness in an elderly patient due to electrolyte changes caused by the taking of laxatives and/or, perhaps, a diuretic) – of which the doctor may or may not be aware. Finally, it must never be dismissed from mind that anyone, even with a long-standing psychiatric history, may well develop a biological illness (with all its sequelae) or, indeed, an additional and unrelated psychological problem of another aetiology.

The mental contribution to the presentation of an illness as a whole may range from being trivial to substantial and might even vary in degree at different times as the symptoms unfold; moreover, it could even be manifest long before the expression of some biological basis becomes clinically recognized.

HISTORICAL CONTEXT

The concept that chemical disorders might underlie disturbances of the mind is not new. In ancient Greece the Hippocratic school believed that such clinical presentations might be caused by abnormalities in the humors of the brain and/or composition of the blood. Nevertheless, it was to wait until 1884 for the founder of modern neurochemistry, J.W.L. Thudichum, to so eloquently express his thoughts and visions as follows: 'Many forms of insanity are unquestionably the external manifestations of the effects upon the brain-substance of poisons fermented within the body, just as the mental aberrations accompanying chronic alcoholic intoxication are the accumulated effects of a relatively simple poison fermented out of the body. These poisons we shall, I have no doubt, be able to isolate after we know the normal chemistry to its uttermost detail. And then will come in their turn the crowning discoveries to which all our efforts must ultimately be directed, namely, the discoveries of the antidotes to the poisons, and to the fermenting causes and processes which produce them'[1].

BIOLOGICAL DISORDERS WITH A PSYCHIATRIC COMPONENT

The biological presentations of the disorders of clinical medicine have, over the years, been well documented in great detail, but there has been noticeably less emphasis on their emotional and/or psychiatric aspects; the reasons for this are many but must, surely, include recognition that these presentations are often dominated by the more obvious and, sometimes, more urgent biological events – which override the mental aspects. Sometimes, the psychological and biological components have a different time scale, one having begun at an earlier or later stage of the illness than the other, thus making it difficult to assuredly associate the two. In other instances the mental symptoms are so minor that, unless they are specifically probed, the patients may not even think to mention them. It may be that of a multitude of minor complaints, each individual one seemingly so trivial and yet collectively causing distress of significant degree, some would be found to have important diagnostic potential. Nevertheless,

2

the patient may be rather wary of 'being seen too readily to complain of trivia' for fear of being regarded as neurotic – hence, important clinical data may never come to light. Not only may such a patient wrongly regard himself as being neurotic, but also this view may be enhanced and seemingly proven by the similarly erroneous views held by close family members, friends, acquaintances and even the medical practitioner.

The precise mode of presentation of any illness is the result of interaction of an individual with the environment; one must, in consequence, be aware of the possible combinations of any or all of the factors so far mentioned as being contributory to construction of such a clinical situation. All the common psychiatric symptoms (e.g. anxiety, depression, phobias, obsessions/compulsions, paranoid feelings, etc.), together with the simple emotional disorders (e.g. feeling irritable, afraid, tired, unhappy, etc.), can be either 'primary' or have a 'secondary' cause – of physical, chemical, biological, psychological or sociological origin. It is those disorders which are secondary to chemical changes that will mainly be elaborated upon in this book (e.g. the depression which may precede or accompany Addison's disease, the anxiety which can be associated with a phaeochromocytoma, and the confusion and aggression which may herald an insulinoma).

PSYCHIATRIC DISORDERS WITH A BIOCHEMICAL BASIS

Psychiatric disorders of biochemical origin may be prime examples of the illusion sometimes created by initially seeing a psychiatric presentation in wrong perspective – and which, in turn, is basically related to the variations in viewpoint of medical practitioners skilled in different disciplines. What may at first seem to be the obvious diagnosis may, quite suddenly, be revealed as being incorrect, particularly when new information has come to light or after one has quietly reflected on the clinical data at hand. The importance of this is well illustrated by depression, previously attributed to some other cause, which quite suddenly becomes a very different situation when the hypercalcaemia of primary hyperparathyroidism is firmly established; the treatment and management would then be re-orientated towards partial parathyroidectomy rather than to the prescribing of pharmacological agents and, perhaps, electroconvulsive therapy (ECT). It is worth drawing attention at this point to the fact that even a number of the standard textbooks of psychiatry do not place sufficient emphasis on the chemical aspects of psychiatric disorders.

Those psychiatric disorders secondary to physical causes (e.g. a cerebral space-occupying lesion, etc.), as opposed to those with a chemical basis (e.g. of biochemical, pharmacological, toxicological, or nutritional origin), will receive only brief mention here. The more formal and florid psychiatric presentations, however, such as schizophrenia and endogenous depression (in which the biochemical disturbances present are as described later in this chapter) will receive more attention; these conditions form entities of their own – but are, nevertheless, rather more 'primary' than the main body of disorders (secondary to biochemical disturbances) to which the reader's attention is particularly directed in Chapters 6, 7 and 10.

A number of case studies, scattered throughout Chapters 6, 7 and 8, some showing interaction between different aetiological factors and others with unexpected sequelae, have been selected in order to illustrate the text in a clinical, practical and, hopefully, instructive way. In each instance, they are placed in the most appropriate portion of the text, but the actual diagnosis does not prominently appear. The reason for this is that in this way the reader can, if he/she so chooses, treat each discussion as a diagnostic challenge, working through the clinical history and investigations before reading the analysis and comments section wherein lies the finally accepted conclusion.

Opportunity will also be taken to refer to the protean manifestations, many of which fall within the field of clinical chemistry, of Munchausen's syndrome – revealing how these curious presentations may confound, confuse or merely puzzle the medical practitioner, often for an inordinately long period of time and involving many costly laboratory investigations, before there is full recognition of what is truly going on (see Chapter 8).

FACTORS INFLUENCING THE BIOCHEMICAL STATE

In a patient with a psychiatric disorder the discovery of what appears to be a well-defined biochemical abnormality should not, necessarily, be attributed solely to the disease process itself[2]. The reasons for this are enumerated as follows:

(1)   The patient may have been institutionalized for many years and might, therefore, have suffered from the infections typical of the life-style of such an environment (e.g. overcrowding, etc.), with consequent secondary effects on the biology and biochemistry of the individual.

(2)   The diet may have lacked quantity, quality and variety for a sufficiently long period of time, on account of the effects on the appetite of mental turmoil, stress and polypharmacy, in sufficient degree to cause nutritional deficiencies (e.g. of energy, proteins, vitamins, etc.).

(3)   The effects of pharmacological therapy, in particular, may profoundly alter certain biochemical processes.

Clearly, any such biochemical changes may be secondary to institutionalization, nutritional deficiencies and pharmacological exposure (including alcohol), in addition to emotional stress accompanying the situation and the disease process itself. Moreover, in an individual patient or in an experimental study group, it is important to remember that any interest shown in the patient may, on its own, be sufficient to motivate improvement in some way. The situation is, therefore, highly complex as all these factors must be foremost in the mind when attempting to interpret the biochemical changes accompanying an apparent beneficial response to therapy.

2
The complexity of the central nervous system

There should be no surprise at finding that the biochemistry, physiology and pathology of the brain is less completely understood than that of any other organ; this becomes clear when one considers just four aspects of cerebral structure and function, namely – the anatomical intricacies of neuronal connections, the high oxygen consumption of cerebral metabolic processes, the constant requirement for energy which is almost entirely from glucose and the complexities of neurotransmission. The brain is, in essence, a large neuroendocrine organ, made up of vast numbers of neurones and synapses, each one being involved in reception (at neurotransmitter receptor sites), processing (the chemical processes taking place within the neuronal axon) and transmission (via the neurotransmitter molecules, receptors and re-uptake mechanisms) of information at each synaptic cleft. The concept that the human brain is the most complex structure in the universe, to our knowledge, seems well founded.

CELLULAR ORGANIZATION

At cell level there is great complexity; there are approximately 10 thousand million neurones in both the cerebral cortex and the cerebellum. In addition, each of these cells makes many connections, with there being up to 60 000 synaptic points on a single cortical neurone, although not all are from different sources[3]. These synaptic points, moreover, can be situated on the cell body of the receiving neurone, on the axon, on the trunk of the dendrites or on the spines which project from them[4]. Furthermore, there are electron microscopic differences, too: excitatory synapses usually have round vesicles and a dense continuous postsynaptic membrane, whereas inhibitory synapses are characterized by flattened synaptic vesicles and discontinuity of the postsynaptic membrane density (Figure 1).

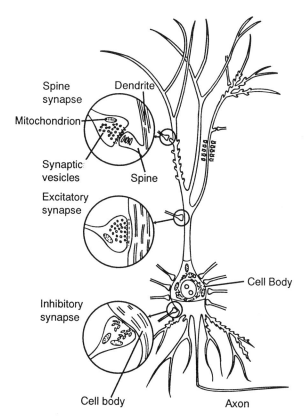

Figure 1 Diagrammatic representation of microstructures involved in neurotransmission

OXYGEN CONSUMPTION

At the physiological level, the brain proves to be the most active energy consumer of all the organs of the body; in keeping with this is its rich blood supply and high oxygen uptake. The adult human brain represents, in fact, just 2% of the total body weight (>2% in babies), but its high oxygen utilization of 50 ml/min equates with 20% of the body's resting oxygen needs[4]. The maximal oxygen consumption by the brain occurs at around six years of age. This ravenous requirement for oxygen is probably essential for maintenance of the ionic gradients across neuronal membranes, on which depend conduction of neural impulses in the many billions of neurones; glucose supplies the energy for these processes. The rate of brain metabolism is much the same both during the day and by night, although there is, perhaps, a slight increase during the rapid eye movement (REM) phase of sleep. If the supply of oxygenated blood to the brain ceases, then consciousness is lost within a period of as little as 10 sec; a similar effect would follow the onset of severe hypoglycaemia of any cause.

ENERGY REQUIREMENT

The constant requirement for energy by the brain is approximately 1700 kJ (405 kcal) per day; this represents approximately 20–25% of the total energy needs of a normal resting adult[5]. The source of energy under normal circumstances is glucose, although the ketones 3-hydroxybutyrate and acetoacetate can be utilized, particularly in conditions of starvation in which they might even replace glucose entirely. Glycogen, too, is present in the brain, but the content of merely 0.1% is insufficient for it to be an important source of energy. There is heavy reliance on the glucose present in the extracellular fluid, because the brain is neither able to store nor synthesize glucose; moreover, the entry of glucose to the brain is not under hormonal control. It is the conversion of approximately 120 g glucose each day to carbon dioxide (CO_2), water (H_2O) and energy that supplies this high energy need. The consequence is that significant hypoglycaemia would drastically impair neuronal function; however, marked hyperglycaemia would also disrupt cerebral function, but in other ways – by causing an osmotic disturbance and also on account of the accompanying metabolic changes in most cases (e.g. metabolic acidosis).

NEUROREGULATION[4,6]

In the central nervous system (CNS), transfer of information from one neurone to another occurs by way of the release of one or more substances from the first neurone, which bind and act at specific receptor sites on the second neurone[4]. This binding, in turn, promotes a sequence of biochemical effects in the second neurone, with consequent physical changes. There are four groups of neuroregulators (Table 1)[6]:

Table 1 Groups of neuroregulators and the compounds involved

Neuroregulator	Compound	Action

Neurotransmitters	Dopamine (DA)
	Noradrenaline (NA)
	Adrenaline (epinephrine)
	Serotonin (5HT)
	Histamine
	Acetylcholine (ACh)
	Inhibitory amino acids
	  gamma-aminobutyric
	  acid (GABA)
	  glycine
	Excitatory amino acids
	  glutamic acid
	  aspartic acid
		These compounds all produce short-lasting rapid-onset, postsynaptic effects (e.g. depolarization close to the point at which they are released)

Neuromodulators	Endorphins Substance P Somatostatin	They modify either by enhancing or lessening the response to a neurotransmitter; they also act close to the point of their release, but do not actually precipitate depolarization
Neurohormones	Vasopressin Angiotensin II (AII)	They are released into the bloodstream; unlike neurotransmitters and neuromodulators, they act remotely on receptors somewhere else in the body. Their effects are, therefore, of later onset, of longer duration and far distant
Neuromediators	Adenosine 3',5'-monophosphate (cyclic AMP cAMP) Guanosine 3',5'-monophosphate (cyclic GMP cGMP)	These compounds act as second messengers at specific sites of synaptic transmission, participating in elicitation of the postsynaptic response to a neurotransmitter

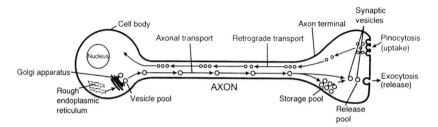

Figure 2 Processes and structures involved in neurotransmission

NEUROTRANSMISSION[4]

Neurotransmitters are synthesized in presynaptic nerve terminals; some, such as ACh and NA, are stored in synaptic vesicles, which lend protection against enzymatic breakdown, which would otherwise occur (Figure 2)[4]. There are many thousands of synaptic vesicles in any one single nerve terminal, each of them containing 10 000–100 000 molecules of neurotransmitter. Following the arrival of a nerve impulse (action potential, AP) there is an increase in permeability to calcium ions, which then enter the nerve terminal leading to fusion of the synaptic vesicles with the membrane of the terminal, thus promoting the release mechanism. The neurotransmitter molecules now enter the synaptic cleft, where they diffuse across the fluid-filled space, moving towards the postsynaptic receptor sites. Postsynaptic biochemical and biophysical changes ensue, the sum of all stimulation and inhibition processes determining the final outcome as to whether or not there will be discharge of the second neurone. The number of neurotransmitters identified now stands in excess of fifty and it is possible that even single neurones might possess the ability to release more than one such substance (Figure 3).

Should a neurotransmitter molecule become bound to its receptor site for too long it would, clearly, act for longer than might be required; hence, there must be a mechanism for its rapid inactivation at that site, in order that there can be precise control of transmission. Acetylcholinesterase (AChE) in the synaptic space hydrolyses ACh; the enzyme can cleave approximately 25 000 molecules of the transmitter per second[4]. NA is inactivated differently – it is released, and then rapidly pumped back inside the cell. The recaptured molecules are

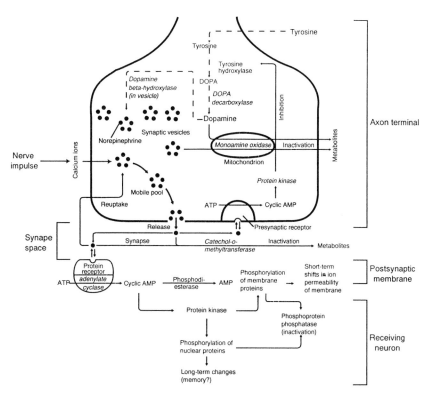

Figure 3 Neurotransmitter synthesis and release

then dealt with in two possible ways, either destruction by catechol-*O*-methyltransferase (COMT) and monoamine oxidase (MAO) in the nerve terminal, or recycled back into the synaptic vesicles; there are re-uptake mechanisms for NA, DA, 5HT and GABA, thus permitting conservation of molecules for several cycles of release and reception[4].

NEUROTRANSMITTER RECEPTION[7]

Apart from the vast number of neurotransmitter substances identified to date, there are now being found an increasing number of receptor subtypes for many of them; the latter are, in turn, linked to ion channels, sometimes involving 'G-proteins' and intracellular second

11

messengers[7]. These ion channels, themselves, reveal further heterogeneity in that their kinetics, their sensitivity to membrane potential and their ion selectivity collectively contribute towards a very complex electrical system. Together, all these biochemical and anatomical pathways at cellular and subcellular level make it possible for neurotransmitters to act on different channels via different receptors, thereby enabling multiple actions by a single cell type. Compound all these factors with the added variations caused by negative feedback and facilitation within and between the different neuronal populations, and one begins to obtain just a glimmer of understanding of the enormous complexity of the situation as a whole.

3
Neurotransmitters, neuronal systems and subcortical nuclei

NEUROTRANSMITTERS

Dopamine (DA)[6,8,9,10]

Biosynthesis

DA is synthesized *via* the conversion of tyrosine to dihydroxyphenyl-alanine (DOPA), involving the enzyme tyrosine hydroxylase, followed by decarboxylation. Dopaminergic neurones lack the enzyme dopamine β-hydroxylase (DBH) and cannot, therefore, convert DA to NA. DA, released from the nerve terminals, is largely recaptured by a re-uptake mechanism (Figure 4).

Degradation

Following re-uptake, DA is metabolized either to dihydroxyphenyl-acetic acid (DOPAC) via oxidative deamination to an intermediate aldehyde compound (involving the enzyme MAO) which is then converted to DOPAC (with the aid of an aldehyde dehydrogenase), or to homovanillic acid (HVA) which is the methoxy derivative of DOPAC (involving the enzyme COMT). The sulfated conjugates of both DOPAC and HVA are ultimately excreted in the urine (Figure 5).

Receptors

DA receptors in the CNS, as in the periphery, are classified as D_1 (which is linked to the enzyme adenyl cyclase) and D_2 (not linked to adenyl cyclase). The presence of the D_2 receptor accounts for the majority of the postsynaptic effects of DA. DA also acts on presynaptic dopaminergic neuronal receptors in both the striatum and the limbic system. It has been postulated that these receptors comprise a third category, i.e. D_3. The antipsychotic activity of the drugs used in

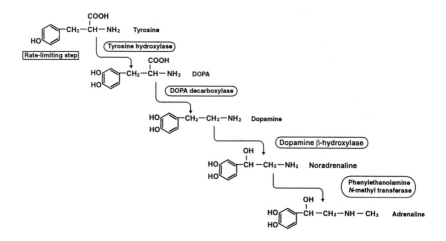

Figure 4 Conversion of tyrosine to dopamine (DA), noradrenaline (NA), and adrenaline. Note: noradrenaline and adrenaline are also known as norepinephrine and epinephrine

schizophrenia (e.g. the phenothiazines) is accounted for by their high affinity for the D_2 receptors, rather than *via* their lesser ability to bind to D_1 sites.

Location

The dopaminergic system comprises a vital part of the extrapyramidal motor control system, dysfunction of which leads to Parkinson's disease as the commonest clinical expression of disorder. In this condition there is deficiency of DA in the striatum causing slowness of movement, in the mesocortical system accounting for muscular rigidity, and in the hypothalamic nuclei causing the tremor. The main dopaminergic pathways are the nigrostriatal pathway (the cell bodies lie in the substantia nigra and the axons end in the corpus striatum), the mesolimbic pathway (the cell bodies lie in the midbrain, the fibres projecting to parts of the limbic system – and to the nucleus accumbens, in particular) and the tuberoinfundibular system (the cell bodies originate in the arcuate nucleus of the hypothalamus, the fibres

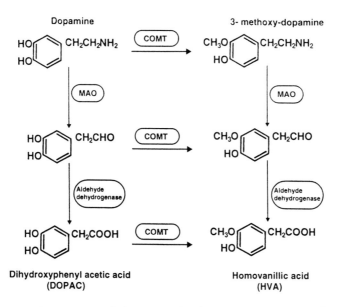

Figure 5 Conversion of dopamine (DA) to its excretory products, dihydroxyphenylacetic acid (DOPAC) and homovanillic acid (HVA)

ending in the pituitary gland, where they are involved in hormone regulation) (Figure 6).

Function

The neurotransmitter DA is fundamental to proper functioning of the basal ganglia and extrapyramidal system. As regards behavioural effects, the 'dopamine hypothesis' (postulating overactivity of the mesolimbic dopaminergic pathways) of schizophrenia has been the most popular one over a number of years. DA is also involved in the control of prolactin (PRL) secretion; its inhibitory influence over PRL release is prevented by many antipsychotic drugs which block DA receptors. Growth hormone (GH) is controlled by DA, too; DA receptor activation increases GH secretion, but inhibits its secretion in pathological situations where there is excessive GH production, as in acromegaly.

Drugs that cause increased DA release in the brain (e.g. levodopa) and DA receptor agonists (e.g. bromocriptine) can both precipitate nausea and vomiting as side effects; DA antagonists (e.g. metoclo-

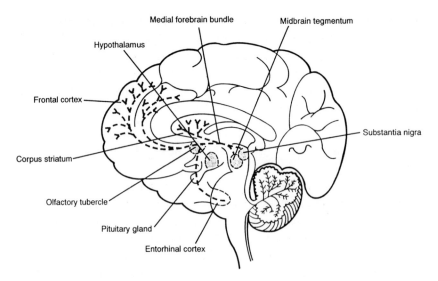

Figure 6 Areas of the brain involved in dopamine (DA) metabolism

pramide), however, are anti-emetic. Deficiency of GABA permits excessive dopaminergic activity in the corpus striatum resulting in onset of Huntington's chorea, on account of the imbalance generated between cholinergic and dopaminergic systems.

Noradrenaline (NA)/norepinephrine[6,8,9,10,11]

Biosynthesis

The amino acid tyrosine, having been actively taken up by adrenergic neurones, is converted to DOPA by means of tyrosine hydroxylase. This enzyme is the rate-limiting step in the biosynthesis of catecholamines; the enzyme is inhibited by NA (in short-term control), long-term control being by means of influence over the rate of biosynthesis of the enzyme itself. DOPA is then converted, with the aid of DOPA decarboxylase, to DA and the latter, in turn, is converted in the synaptic vesicles by means of DBH to NA. Conversion of the latter to adrenaline occurs by means of the enzyme phenylethanolamine *N*-methyltransferase (PNMT) in the adrenal medulla and also in certain restricted parts of the brain. The majority of NA is stored in the nerve terminals in synaptic vesicles, with a small additional amount being free in the cytoplasm. Following arrival of the nerve impulse NA is released, together with adenosine triphosphate (ATP) and chromogranin (a protein), the three substances having already formed a complex within the vesicle; this complex formation serves the purpose not only of preventing NA leakage from the vesicle into the nerve terminal but also in keeping down the osmolality of the vesicle contents (Figure 4).

Degradation

Catecholamine degradation is enzymatically controlled by MAO and COMT. The metabolism of NA is different within the CNS compared with the periphery; this is because the influence of MAO is greater intra-neuronally, with the result that NA is deaminated to 3,4-dihydroxy-phenylglycoaldehyde (DOPGAL). This aldehyde is, in turn, reduced by aldehyde reductase (AR) to the corresponding glycol, 3,4-dihy-droxyphenylethylene glycol (DOPEG), within the neurone. The DOPEG is then converted by means of COMT to 3-methoxy-4-hydroxy-phenylethylene glycol (MOPEG) which is excreted in the urine, after conjugation with sulfate, as MOPEG sulfate. For comparison, the end product in the periphery is vanillylmandelic acid (VMA) (Figure 7).

Receptors

As in the peripheral nervous system, the CNS contains four subtypes of adrenergic receptors, these being designated α_1, α_2, β_1 and β_2. Within the CNS, activation of α_2 receptors causes inhibition of NA and ACh release respectively, from adrenergic and cholinergic autonomic nerve terminals, whereas activators of β_1 receptors leads to increased release of NA from adrenergic terminals. In the body as a whole, the adrenoreceptor subtypes of α_1, α_2, β_1 and β_2 are functional in a variety of other ways. Stimulation of the α_1 receptors is responsible for smooth muscle contraction in a number of organs including blood vessels and bronchi, although there is relaxation of gastrointestinal smooth muscle; α_2 receptor stimulation causes constriction of blood vessels; β_1 receptors are found mainly in the heart where stimulation causes an increase both in rate and force of contraction but in the gastrointestinal tract, there is smooth muscle relaxation and stimulation of β_2 receptors

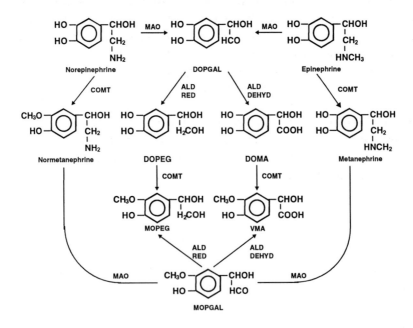

Figure 7 The degradation of catecholamines

is responsible for initiating smooth muscle relaxation in several organs, bronchodilatation and vasodilatation.

Location

The locus coeruleus is a small collection of neurones, located within the pons, comprising the main noradrenergic nucleus and producing NA as neurotransmitter. Fibres from the locus coeruleus are distributed widely in the cerebral cortex, striatum, thalamus and cerebellum. NA is present in moderate amounts in most regions of the brain, but is particularly abundant in the hypothalamus and parts of the limbic system (e.g. the amygdala and the dentate gyrus of the hippocampus).

Function

The noradrenergic system is powerfully involved in the determination of mood, dysfunction equating with the 'functional' disorders of depression, mania and anxiety. The 'noradrenergic hypothesis' of depression refers to the inability of depressed patients to produce sufficient NA in some parts of the brain for neuronal transmission; mania could be associated with excessive activity or sensitivity of this system. The pleasurable experience promoted by stimulation of an electrode implanted in the region of the noradrenergic projection from the locus coeruleus to the limbic and cortical areas of an animal (and which leads to repeated self-stimulation via a switch it can learn to control) makes the noradrenergic system a 'reward' system. Noradrenergic pathway stimulation also produces arousal and alertness; patients with severe depression are lethargic and unresponsive to external stimuli.

Adrenaline/epinephrine[6,9,10,11]

Biosynthesis

The biosynthesis of adrenaline occurs by way of the sequence tyrosine, DOPA, DA, NA, and adrenaline (Figure 4).

Degradation

Enzymatic degradation parallels that of the other catecholamines (Figure 7).

Receptors

Receptor sites for adrenaline are as for NA (i.e. α and β receptors).

Location

Adrenaline is the major hormone of the adrenal medulla but is also a neurotransmitter in the CNS, although it is not well represented there. However, adrenaline-containing neurones are found in the medullary reticular formation, with connections being made to some pontine and diencephalic nuclei, and with some extending as far as the paraventricular nuclei (of the dorsal midline thalamus).

Function

Adrenaline is the 'fight, flight, and fright' hormone, involved in the functioning of the sympathetic nervous system; it also serves the above-mentioned neural pathways in the CNS.

Serotonin (5-hydroxytryptamine, 5HT)[6,8,12–14]

Biosynthesis

Tryptophan is obtained from dietary protein, its transport into the brain being facilitated by insulin secreted in response to dietary carbohydrates. The reason for this is that tryptophan competes with phenylalanine, tyrosine, leucine, isoleucine and valine which are the other large neutral amino acids (LNAA), the concentration of these in the blood being reduced by the action of insulin on skeletal muscle – thus increasing the tryptophan : LNAA ratio. Tryptophan is then taken up by active transport into the neurones where it is hydroxylated by means of tryptophan hydroxylase (the rate-limiting enzyme in the process) to 5-hydroxytryptophan (5HTP). The latter is then decarboxylated to 5HT which, following release from the neurones, is recovered by a re-uptake mechanism (Figure 8).

Degradation

Degradation of 5HT to 5-hydroxyindoleacetaldehyde occurs by way of MAO; most is dehydrogenated by aldehyde dehydrogenase to 5-hydroxyindoleacetic acid (5HIAA), which is excreted in the urine.

Receptors

An increasingly complex series of 5HT receptors is being identified. Presynaptic 5HT uptake sites and receptors, designated $5HT_1$ (and further subdivided into $5HT_{1A}$, $5HT_{1B}$, $5HT_{1C}$, $5HT_{1D}$), $5HT_2$, $5HT_3$ and possibly $5HT_4$, have been identified by means of pharmacological studies. In many neurones 5HT co-exists with other neurotransmitters – and the system, as a whole, interacts in a complex manner with many other neurotransmitter and neuropeptide systems.

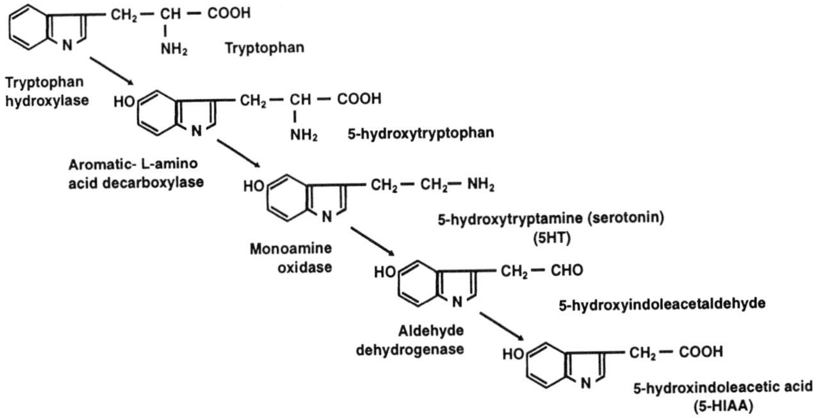

Figure 8 The synthesis and degradation of serotonin (5HT)

Location

5HT is the neurotransmitter of the serotoninergic system, an anatomically diverse system with pathways which follow very closely those of the noradrenergic system, but which are very different from those of dopaminergic distribution. The serotoninergic system comprises several large clusters of cells located in the pons and upper medulla (i.e. the cell bodies of the dorsal and median raphe). The rostral nuclei project to innervate the cerebral cortex, hippocampus, limbic areas and hypothalamus, whereas the more caudal nuclei project to the medulla and spinal cord.

Function

The physiological functions in which the serotoninergic system is involved include sleep, appetite, nociception, diurnal rhythmicity, neuroendocrine regulation and mood. At the level of consciousness there is also the suggestion that rational thought processes arise, using previously stored information, with the aid of the serotoninergic system. Serotoninergic projections innervating the hypothalamus influence the secretions of several anterior pituitary hormones. There is evidence that 5HT may serve as the final common pathway by which other neurotransmitters act in controlling secretion of GH.

The whole system may be severely affected in patients with major mood disorders, in which the use of serotoninergic drugs may be able to either alleviate or prevent such changes of mood. Those antidepressants with more specificity for the serotoninergic system have significant advantages over others; this appears to be related to their anti-obsessional effects rather than with the ability to alleviate concomitant depression. Partial $5HT_{1A}$ agonists (e.g. buspirone and ipsapirone) are effective anxiolytic agents according to preliminary evidence. Selective 5HT uptake inhibitors and $5HT_2$ antagonists may be more effective in relieving the depression of patients where anxiety is a prominent feature than in those with psychotic depression. The $5HT_2$ receptors, in particular, are the sites of action of many hallucinogenic drugs, e.g. lysergic acid diethylamide (LSD). The action of the compound clozapine, used in the therapy of patients with schizophrenia where 'negative' symptoms (e.g. emotional flattening, lack of volition and a decrease in motor activity) predominate and who fail to respond to neuroleptics, may be related to its effect on $5HT_2$ receptors.

Histamine

Biosynthesis

Decarboxylation of histidine to histamine requires the enzyme histidine decarboxylase.

Degradation

Histamine is mainly converted to methylhistamine by histamine-*N*-methyltransferase and then to methylimidazoleacetic acid with the aid of MAO. A small amount of histamine is converted to imidazoleacetic acid by diamine oxidase (histaminase).

Receptors

There are three receptors for histamine – H_1, H_2 and H_3; all of these are found in peripheral tissues and in the CNS. The H_1 receptors activate phospholipase C, H_2 receptors increase the cAMP concentration within cells and the H_3 receptors, being mainly presynaptic, mediate inhibition of histamine (and other neurotransmitters) release by way of a G protein.

Location

The tuberomammillary nucleus of the posterior hypothalamus contains the cell bodies of histaminergic neurones; their axons project to many parts of the cerebral cortex and spinal cord.

Function

The histaminergic system has an uncertain function but does involve the processes of arousal, sexual behaviour, drinking and setting pain thresholds; histamine is also involved in regulating secretion of anterior pituitary hormones and blood pressure.

Acetylcholine (ACh)[6,8,10,15]

Biosynthesis

Acetyl coenzyme A (acetyl CoA), which is required for the synthesis of ACh, is derived either from pyruvate (catalysed by pyruvate dehydrogenase) or, alternatively, is synthesized via acetate and ATP to form acetyl AMP; the latter, in the presence of coenzyme A (CoA), is enzymically converted to acetyl CoA. It is the acetylation of choline with acetyl CoA, in the presence of choline acetyltransferase (CAT) following choline uptake by the nerve terminals, that is the final step in ACh synthesis. The rate-limiting step in the whole process is choline transportation, the regulation of which depends on the rate at which ACh is released. Most of the ACh formed is stored in the synaptic vesicles.

Degradation

Following release into the synaptic cleft, after arrival of the nerve impulse, ACh diffuses to combine with the postsynaptic receptors. However, some ACh is hydrolysed in the immediate vicinity of the nerve endings by AChE – to choline and acetic acid. AChE is found not only in the neurones but also at neuromuscular junctions and in some other tissues, too.

Receptors

As in the periphery, both nicotinic and muscarinic receptors are represented in the brain, either of which can mediate the usually excitatory influence to the next neurone after binding with ACh. However, the muscarinic rather than the nicotinic receptors are responsible for most of the behavioural effects associated with cholinergic pathways.

Location

The corpus striatum has the highest content of ACh, AChE and CAT of any structure in the brain; disease of this structure is the basis of Parkinson's disease and Huntington's chorea. In a normal individual the release of ACh from the striatum is inhibited by the presence of DA; lack of DA leads to cholinergic hyperactivity with the result of Parkinson's disease, whereas deficiency of GABA leads to excessive dopaminergic activity resulting in Huntington's chorea. It is the imbalance between cholinergic and dopaminergic activity which creates the symptomatology. Several neuronal pathways in the brain and spinal cord utilize ACh as their neurotransmitter. Many varied mental and motor activities possess a cholinergic component. The basal forebrain cholinergic neurones project to a number of structures including the hippocampus. ACh is well represented in the cerebral cortex, the midbrain and brainstem, but is poorly represented in the cerebellum.

Function

Learning and short-term memory involve cholinergic pathways. Dementia, both senile and presenile, characterized by loss both of memory and other intellectual abilities, is accompanied by functional disturbance of the cholinergic system. In a wide range of clinical disorders, where dementia is a feature, there is degeneration of the forebrain cholinergic system (e.g. Alzheimer's disease, etc.). Cortical and hippocampal CAT and AChE activities are considerably reduced in senile dementia, but not in patients with depression or schizophrenia.

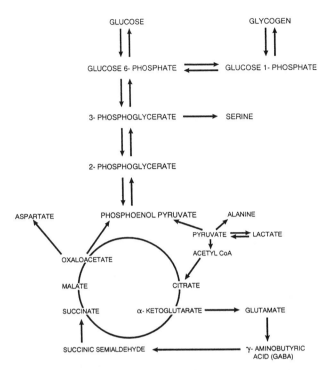

Figure 9 Some important pathways of glucose metabolism in the mammalian brain

Gamma-aminobutyric acid (GABA)[6,8]

Biosynthesis

The conversion of glutamate to GABA, involving the enzyme glutamic acid decarboxylase (GAD) and requiring the assistance of pyridoxal phosphate, is the major source of this neurotransmitter (Figure 9).

Degradation

Active uptake by GABA-ergic neurones is the initial step in removing the GABA released previously into the synaptic cleft. Then follows conversion to succinic semialdehyde during a transamination reaction involving GABA-transaminase (GABA-T), during which process the amino group of GABA is transferred to α-oxoglutaric acid, yielding glutamate.

Receptors

$GABA_A$ and $GABA_B$ are now established as the two types of receptors for GABA. It is by way of increased chloride permeability of the post-synaptic membrane that $GABA_A$ functions; there is, in consequence, reduced depolarization following the action of an excitatory neuro-transmitter. $GABA_B$ effects are, in some neurones, due to inhibition of the calcium channel, thus accounting for a decrease in the neurotrans-mitter released. $GABA_A$ receptors possess at least four binding sites. In addition to the binding site for (i) GABA, there are binding sites for: (ii) benzodiazepines, anxiolytics and beta-carbolines, (iii) barbiturates and (iv) convulsants (e.g. picrotoxin). Benzodiazepine compounds bind to the $GABA_A$ site causing enhanced GABA binding, hence leading to marked neuronal inhibition. Potentiation of the effects of GABA on $GABA_A$ receptors is also caused by barbiturates, but less selectively. It is possible that endogenous anxiolytics or anxiogenic molecules exist in the body. This would be a reasonable expectation when one consid-ers that following identification of opiate receptors in the brain it was not long before endogenous opiates were discovered. Patients suffer-ing from chronic alcoholism have a decrease in the accessory sites on the $GABA_A$ receptor to which benzodiazepines bind.

Location

GABA is predominantly found in the short interneurones of the cerebral cortex, having widespread and largely uniform cerebral representation. GABA-ergic tracts extending to the striatum and cerebellum are the only long tracts using GABA as neurotransmitter.

Function

GABA, and to a lesser extent glycine, are the inhibitory amino acid transmitters of the CNS. Deficiency of GABA permits excessive activity of the dopaminergic system in the corpus striatum, causing Huntington's chorea. In this disorder there is neurodegeneration of the GABA-ergic projections from the corpus striatum to the lateral globus pallidus or substantia nigra as the basis of the imbalance between dopaminergic and cholinergic systems. It is the tight binding of the benzodiazepine compounds to an accessory site on the $GABA_A$

receptor that permits facilitation of GABA binding, thus enhancing pharmacological activity.

Glycine (Gly)[6,8]

Biosynthesis

Conversion of glyoxylate and glutamate to glycine occurs by way of a reaction involving the enzyme glycine transaminase, during which process α-oxoglutarate is also formed.

Degradation

The carbon skeleton may be oxidized completely to CO_2 by conversion to pyruvate *via* serine, condensation with succinyl CoA to yield α-amino-β-ketoa dipic acid and condensation with acetyl CoA to form α-amino-β-keto butyric acid. The pathway to pyruvate is quantitatively of little importance. Glycine may also be catabolized to glyoxylate – but this too, seems to be quantitatively minimal.

Receptors

Important evidence that glycine is a neurotransmitter comes from the observation that the convulsant compound, strychnine, blocks the normal synaptic inhibitory effect of glycine.

Location

Glycine is present in high concentration in the grey matter of the spinal cord, particularly the ventral quadrant. It is also present in the reticular formation in the brainstem.

Function

Glycine and GABA are the two inhibitory neurotransmitters of the CNS. Glycine possesses an inhibitory role in the spinal cord at the site where the spinal interneurones synapse with motor neurones. It is also likely to be the inhibitory transmitter for the reticular formation, but not the cuneate nucleus. It is of note that following ischaemic degeneration of the ventral quadrant interneurones of the spinal cord there is parallel reduction in glycine concentration.

Glutamate[6,8]

Biosynthesis

Glutamic acid is a dicarboxylic amino acid. Interconversion of glutamate and α-oxoglutarate occurs with the aid of the enzyme glutamate dehydrogenase. During reductive amination of α-ketoglutarate by NH_4^+ there is utilization of nicotinamide adenine dinucleotide phosphate (reduced) (NADPH) (Figure 9).

Degradation

Glutamate is degraded by glutamate dehydrogenase in the presence of nicotinamide adenine dinucleotide (oxidized) (NAD) and nicotinamide adenine dinucleotide phosphate (oxidized) (NADP) to form α-ketoglutarate. Glutamate is also decarboxylated by glutamic acid decarboxylase to form GABA.

Receptors

The different glutamate receptors are each coupled to a different effector mechanism. N-methyl-D-aspartate (NMDA) is a glutamate analogue which binds firmly with the NMDA receptor, to which glutamate also binds; the associated ion channels are very sensitive to blocking by the presence of magnesium ions. Many CNS synapses involving glutamate are of this category; excitatory interneurones of the spinal cord use NMDA receptors, but not so for the primary afferent neurones. The QUIS receptor responds to quisqualic acid and the KAI receptor is sensitive to kainic acid. All the three receptors mentioned (NMDA, QUIS and KAI) are excitatory; NMDA receptors mediate the slower excitatory synaptic responses, whereas QUIS and KAI receptors are involved in faster transmission.

Location

Glutamate is widely and uniformly represented in high concentration throughout the CNS; in particular, it is well established as a neurotransmitter in the olfactory tract, hippocampus and corticostriate pathways.

Function

Most neurones exposed to glutamate respond by depolarization and excitation on account of increased membrane conductance to sodium and other cations. Glutamate is, therefore, an excitatory amino acid neurotransmitter; aspartate acts similarly. The NMDA receptor is of importance in neuronal degeneration.

Aspartate[6,8]

Biosynthesis

The carbon skeleton of glucose is the basis of aspartate (and of glutamate) manufacture. It is from oxaloacetate, in Krebs tricarboxylic acid cycle, that aspartate is formed (Figure 9) by transamination.

Degradation

Asparagine is formed from aspartate, catalysed by asparagine synthetase. However, asparagine can be catalysed by asparaginase to aspartate which, in turn, can revert to oxaloacetate via a transaminase reaction.

Receptors

Multiple subtypes of receptors for the excitatory amino acid neurotransmitters have been revealed using synthetic agonists and antagonists; these have been discussed above (see Glutamate, page 28). Less is written in the literature regarding aspartate action.

Location

Aspartate, as is also the case with glutamate (the other excitatory amino acid neurotransmitter) and GABA (an inhibitory amino acid neurotransmitter), is present in the cerebral cortex in high amounts.

Function

Aspartate is an excitatory amino acid neurotransmitter, acting very much like glutamate in mediating fast excitatory synaptic responses.

NEUROMODULATORS

Opioid peptides[16]

Biosynthesis

More than 18 opioid peptides have now been identified; each can be assigned to one of three distinct families of compounds, namely – enkephalins, endorphins and dynorphins. These peptide structures have precursor polypeptide compounds in which they reside, and from which they can be cleaved and released as free entities; moreover, these precursors include both prepro- and pro- forms.

Pro-enkephalin is precursor of the two closely related pentapeptides, met-enkephalin and leu-enkephalin. *Pro-opiomelanocortin* (POMC) is precursor of endorphins and other shorter peptides; it contains the sequences of (and can be converted to) melanocyte-stimulating hormone (γ-MSH), adrenocorticotrophic hormone (ACTH) and β-lipotrophin (β-LPH). ACTH (1–39) is a 39 amino acid polypeptide which contains within it the sequence of α-MSH (1–13) and corticotrophin-like intermediate lobe peptide (CLIP) (18–39). β-LPH (1–91) is a polypeptide compound of 91 amino acids and contains within its sequence γ-LPH (1–58) and β-endorphin (61–91). γ-LPH, in turn, contains within its sequence β-MSH (41–58), whereas β-endorphin contains the sequence γ-endorphin (61–77); both β-MSH and β-endorphin form an entity. α-Endorphin (61–76), resides within the γ-endorphin polypeptide. Hence, met-enkephalin (61–65) is a pentapeptide sequence at the N terminal of β, γ and α-endorphin. However, although β-endorphin does contain the amino acid sequence of met-enkephalin this is not the way it is formed biologically; the source of met-enkephalin, as has already been explained, is pro-enkephalin. *Pro-dynorphin* yields at least 7 peptides that contain the sequence of leu-enkephalin; these enclude dynorphin A (1–17), which can be further cleaved to dynorphin A (1–8) and dynorphin B

30

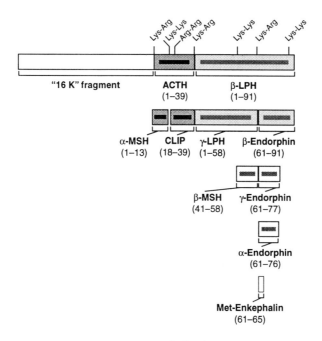

Figure 10 Schematic representation of the bovine precursor molecule indicating an NH$_2$-terminal fragment, followed by ACTH (1–39), which is followed by the β-lipotrophic hormone (β-LPH, β-lipotrophin) (1–91) sequence

(1–13), in addition to α- and β-neoendorphin (which themselves differ by only one amino acid from each other) (Figure 10).

Degradation

Degradation of the precursor molecules, yielding smaller peptide sequences, has been documented above. The enkephalin molecule is split at the gly–phe bond by enkephalinase A, at the gly–gly bond by enkephalinase B and at tyr–gly bonds by aminopeptidase.

Receptors

Opioid peptides bind to opiate receptors in the brain and gastrointestinal tract; to date three receptors have been identified, namely μ, δ and κ. The natural ligands for these receptors are as follows: β-endorphin for the μ receptor, enkephalins for the δ receptor and dynorphins for the κ receptor.

Location

Pro-enkephalin is present throughout the brain and also within the adrenal glands. The enkephalins, too, are identified in the brain, particularly in the substantia gelatinosa, and in the nerve endings of the gastrointestinal tract. POMC is formed in the cell bodies of neurones in the arcuate nuclei from which they project to the thalamus and various parts of the brain stem; it is also formed in the pituitary gland. Pro-dynorphin is formed mainly within the neurones of the hypothalamus, the limbic system and the brain stem.

Function

Activation of opioid receptors inhibits synaptic transmission in the pathways of pain. Enkephalin appears to function in synaptic transmission; injection of these into the brain stem leads to analgesic activity and decreased gastrointestinal motility. Following stimulation of the μ opiate receptors there is euphoria, analgesia, depression of respiration and constipation. Stimulation of κ opiate receptors causes sedation, dysphoria, analgesia and diuresis. Stimulation of the δ opiate receptors leads to analgesia. Activation of the μ receptor increases potassium conductance, thus causing hyperpolarisation of central neurones and primary afferents. Activation of κ receptors closes calcium ion channels, as also does activation of the δ receptors. Calcium channel inactivation leads to reduced neurotransmitter release in the presynaptic membrane.

NEURONAL SYSTEMS AND SUBCORTICAL NUCLEI[17]

It will be necessary to provide a brief account of the main CNS structures and pathways (within the context of the biological basis of both emotions and psychiatric illnesses) prior to discussing the neurotransmission involvements of each. This is because these structures are integrally involved in forming the anatomical and physiological basis of emotional experience. All this will be antecedent to providing an account of the essential neurosecretory abnormalities identified within the brains of patients suffering from the major psychoses. The brain areas to receive special mention are the cerebral cortex, basal ganglia, limbic system, hypothalamus and reticular activating system (RAS).

Cerebral cortex[6,17–19]

Anatomy

Besides the well established motor and sensory areas of the cerebral cortex, there are also association areas which integrate, via interconnecting neuronal pathways, the functions of the various cortical areas, e.g. frontal, parietal, temporal and hippocampal.

Neural connections

Innervation of the cerebral cortex is from several sources: cholinergically – from cell bodies beneath the basal ganglia; noradrenergically – from the locus coeruleus in the floor of the fourth ventricle; serotoninergically – from cell bodies in the median raphe nuclei in the pons; and dopaminergically – from extensive cortical and subcortical connections starting in the basal ganglia and going to parts of the frontal and temporal cortex (Figure 11).

Neurotransmission

In the cerebral cortex, the neuropeptides, i.e. somatostatin, corticotrophin releasing factor (CRF), vasoactive intestinal peptide (VIP), cholecystokinin (CCK), neurotensin (NT) and substance P, have all been detected immunochemically within cortical neurones – but not, apparently, within the large pyramidal neurones which project to extracortical sites. On the other hand, the excitatory amino acid neurotransmitters (i.e. glutamic acid and aspartic acid), and the inhibitory amino acids (e.g. GABA) are well represented in high concentrations in the cerebral cortex (Figure 12).

Function

Functions of the cerebral cortex comprise perception, the control of movement and, at even higher level, all the intricacies and ramifications of communication by means of the use of language. However, in addition

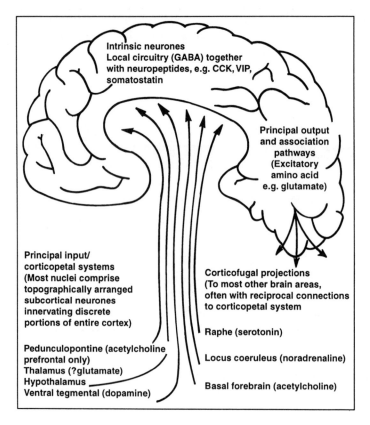

Figure 11 Neurotransmission within the cerebral cortex (after Perry, E.K. (1991). Neurotransmitters and diseases of the brain. *British Journal of Hospital Medicine*, **45**, 73–83)

to these more regionalized functions there are others which are based on wider integration of many cortical areas with RAS connections – namely, the state of wakefulness and its accompanying awareness.

Basal ganglia[17,20]

Anatomy

The basal ganglia are a group of subcortical nuclei located beneath the lateral ventricles. The major ones are the caudate nucleus and putamen (together comprising the striatum), the globus pallidum (possessing

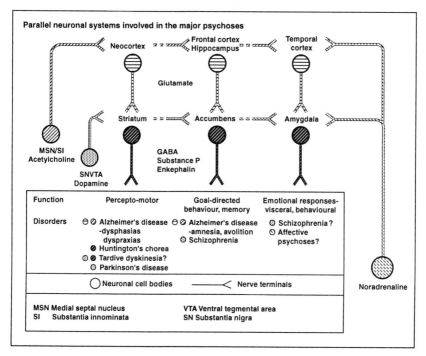

Figure 12 Brain structures, neurotransmitters and psychiatric states (Reproduced from Deakin, B. (1987). Biological Mechanisms in the Major Psychiatric Syndromes. *Medicine*, **43**, 1764–9, by kind permission of the Medicine Group (Journals) Ltd.)

both internal and external segments), the subthalamic nuclei, the substantia nigra and related brain stem structures; there are extensive cortical and subcortical connections. The striatum extends ventrally and medially towards the nucleus accumbens. It also extends posteriorly, turning inferiorly and anteriorly towards the temporal lobe and amygdala (Figure 13).

Neural connections

Glutamatergic innervation of the basal ganglia, nucleus accumbens and amygdala is received from appropriate parts of the cerebral cortex (i.e. the neocortex, frontal cortex and hippocampus, and the temporal cortex, respectively). Dopaminergic terminals arise from cells of the substantia nigra. The mesolimbic dopaminergic area is the probable

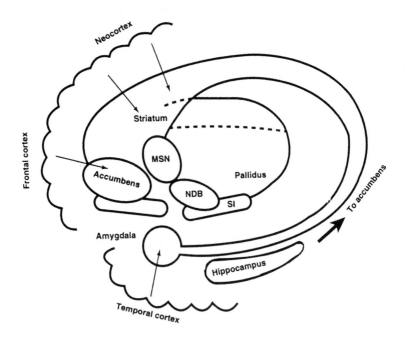

MSN: Medial septal nucleus   SI : Substantia Innominata
NDS: Nucleus of the diagonal band

Figure 13 The anatomical relationships and connections of basal ganglia structures. (Reproduced from Deakin, B. (1987). Biological Mechanisms in the Major Psychiatric Syndromes. *Medicine*, **43**, 1764–9, by kind permission of The Medicine Group (Journals) Ltd.)

site at which neuroleptic drugs act to produce their antipsychotic action. Mesolimbic DA-containing neurones also contain CCK and NT, which act as co-transmitters with DA; these neuropeptides modulate the dopaminergic system locally. Serotoninergic innervation comes to the basal ganglia from the raphe nuclei. ACh, GABA, substance P and enkephalin are all found in the efferent neuronal outflow from the basal ganglia, nucleus accumbens and amygdala (Figure 13).

Neurotransmission

The striatum, amygdala and nucleus accumbens possess abundant ACh (largely on account of the interneuronal cholinergic connections within the basal ganglia) and DA (because of the plentiful dopaminergic innervation). Neuropeptides, such as CCK, NT and thyrotrophin-releasing hormone (TRH), are well represented in the nucleus accumbens; several neuropeptides are also found in the amygdala in high amounts.

Function

The basal ganglia, although mainly involved with modulation of motor activity, also have some behavioural functions. The nucleus accumbens, in particular, is functionally closely related to the limbic system, being involved with incentive and reward. The amygdala, anatomically and functionally part of the limbic system, is involved in emotional response.

Limbic system[6,21–23]

Anatomy

The limbic system is now regarded as an assembly of many specific areas of the brain (Figure 14). It has 'grown' over the years, having been first described by P. Broca in 1878; he referred to 'le grand lobe limbique' which was located on the medial wall of the cerebral hemisphere. In 1901, S. Raman y Cajal referred to the hippocampal– fornix system, which was a portion of the limbic lobe, and confirmed, contrary to previous supposition, that it was unrelated to the neighbouring olfactory apparatus, the implication being that it perhaps served some other function(s). In 1937, J.W. Papez postulated that the cingulate, hippocampus, fornix, mammillary bodies, anterior thalamus and cingulate structures formed a 'circuit' which was fundamental to emotional experience and the expression thereof. In 1934, P. Bard provided evidence to show that the hypothalamus was involved in the 'rage response'. In 1948, P.I. Yakovlev added to this 'medial system' group of structures another group called the 'basolateral components', comprising the orbitofrontal, insular and anterior temporal lobe cortical

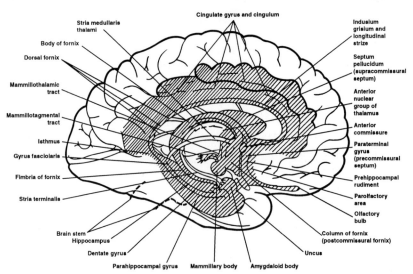

Figure 14 The limbic system in relation to other cerebral structures (from *Gray's Anatomy* with permission from Churchill Livingstone)

region, the amygdala and the dorsomedial nucleus of the thalamus. This assembly, comprising portions of the frontal, temporal and hippo-campal areas of the cerebral cortex, is now referred to as the limbic system. A large part of the limbic system is located within the confines of the temporal lobes (Figure 15).

Neural connections

The reticular system, although anatomically distinct from the limbic system, is physiologically part of it; the two structures communicate by way of the median forebrain bundle. Short neural pathways connect the reticular system, the thalamus, the hypothalamus and most of the contiguous areas of the basal portion of the brain.

Neurotransmission

NA is abundant in parts of the limbic system, particularly the central nucleus of the amygdala and the dentate gyrus of the hippocampus. DA is well represented, too, in the form of long projections of dopaminergic neurones – between the substantia nigra and ventral tegmentum and targets in the limbic zones of the cerebral cortex and

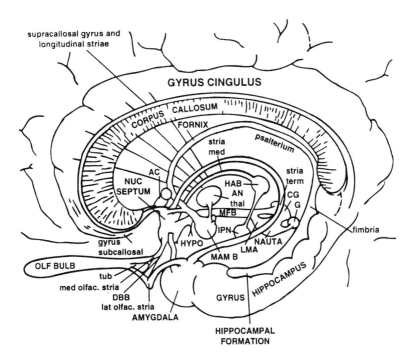

Figure 15 The limbic system and its connections

other major regions of the limbic system. Serotoninergic neurones project to the limbic system from the dorsal and median raphe in the brainstem. The amygdala possesses large quantities of neuropeptides.

Function

The limbic system possesses a central role in emotional experience, behaviour and memory. The hypothalamus, reticular system (in the brainstem) and basal ganglia (extrapyramidal system), although not strictly part of the limbic system anatomically are, nevertheless, closely integrated with it (and each other) functionally; they all exert influence on behaviour. The nucleus accumbens, in particular, serves as a bridge, permitting there to be limbic influence over motor function.

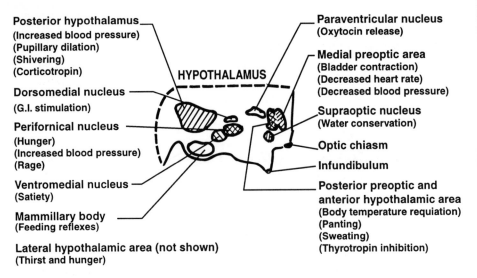

Posterior hypothalamus
(Increased blood pressure)
(Pupillary dilation)
(Shivering)
(Corticotropin)

HYPOTHALAMUS

Dorsomedial nucleus
(G.I. stimulation)

Perifornical nucleus
(Hunger)
(Increased blood pressure)
(Rage)

Ventromedial nucleus
(Satiety)

Mammillary body
(Feeding reflexes)

Lateral hypothalamic area (not shown)
(Thirst and hunger)

Paraventricular nucleus
(Oxytocin release)

Medial preoptic area
(Bladder contraction)
(Decreased heart rate)
(Decreased blood pressure)

Supraoptic nucleus
(Water conservation)

Optic chiasm

Infundibulum

Posterior preoptic and
anterior hypothalamic area
(Body temperature requiation)
(Panting)
(Sweating)
(Thyrotropin inhibition)

Figure 16 The hypothalamus – anatomy, physiology and behavioural aspects (reproduced with permission from Guyton, A.C. (1981) *Textbook of Medical Physiology*, sixth edition, W.B. Saunders Co.)

Hypothalamus[21,24–28]

Anatomy

Although the hypothalamus is located in close proximity to the limbic system, the two structures being functionally integrally related, it is convenient from anatomical and physiological viewpoints to consider it separately. Lying in the middle of the limbic system, the hypothalamus is surrounded by the various subcortical structures of that system – including the preoptic area, the septum, the paraolfactory area, the epithalamus, the anterior nuclei of the thalamus, certain parts of the basal ganglia, the hippocampus and the amygdala. The control centres of the hypothalamus comprise the posterior hypothalamus, dorsomedial nucleus, perifornical nucleus, ventromedial nucleus, mammillary body, lateral hypothalamic area, paraventricular nucleus, medial preoptic area, supraoptic nucleus, the preoptic area and the anterior hypothalamic area (Figure 16).

Neural connections

Short neural pathways connect the hypothalamus with the reticular system, the thalamus and most of the contiguous areas of the basal part of the brain. The hypothalamus comprises the major output pathway of the limbic system.

Neurotransmission

Various neurotransmitter systems determine hormonal secretions from the hypothalamus and pituitary gland; neurotransmitters involved include 5HT, DA, NA and ACh.

Function

Apart from hunger, satiety, thirst and rage, which are all behavioural functions, the hypothalamus is involved in blood pressure control, heart rate determination, body temperature regulation and hormonal control. It is by way of the reticular system in the brainstem that many of the behavioural functions of the hypothalamus are elicited.

Reticular activating system (RAS)[18,29]

Anatomy

The RAS is a physiological concept rather than an anatomical one. The reticular formation, in which the RAS is contained, comprises neurones located within the brainstem, extending from the medulla to the posterior diencephalon.

Neural connections

Neurones of the reticular formation have long-ranging rostrocaudal connections; the majority project to the cerebral cortex *via* a relay system sited in the thalamus.

Neurotransmission

Cholinergic nerve fibres provide connections from the midbrain to the upper brainstem, thalamus and cerebral cortex; these pathways mediate arousal. Noradrenergic neurones in the locus coeruleus project to the cerebral cortex, as also do serotoninergic neurones in the raphe nucleus of the pons. Both ACh and NA are well established in influencing arousal; 5HT and NA serve in the sleep–wake cycle. Amphetamine compounds possess an alerting function, by way of catecholamine release.

Function

The neurones in the area ranging from the rostral part of the pons to the caudal portion of the diencephalon have particular involvement with maintaining the state of wakefulness.

NEUROTRANSMITTER INVOLVEMENT IN DISEASE STATES[30–32]

Several groups of clinical disorders, e.g. those of movement, mood and intellect, possess important underlying neurotransmitter involvements of varying degree and at different locations within the CNS. Neuro-transmitter abnormalities are implicated in disorders of movement (e.g. Parkinson's disease, Huntington's disease, motor neurone disease, etc.), disorders of mood (e.g. unipolar depression, manic–depressive illness, anxiety, etc.) and diseases involving the intellect (e.g. Alzheimer's disease, Jakob–Creutzfeldt disease, Hallerworden–Spatz disease, Lewy body dementia, Wernicke's encephalopathy, Korsakoff psychosis, schizophrenia, etc.). In addition, neurotransmitter involvement has been implicated in many other disorders, such as coma, head injury, cerebral infarction, epilepsy, alcoholism and the mental retardation states of metabolic origin seen particularly in childhood (Chapter 10).

There is often, nevertheless, an overlap between different groups of disorders (e.g. depression may sometimes accompany Parkinson's disease or Alzheimer's disease and schizophrenia may co-exist with Parkinson's disease); many other clinical examples will be seen from time to time. All these disorders of mood and intellect will be elaborated upon later (Chapter 4). Moreover, it was once assumed that disease processes involve essentially only one neurotransmitter substance – but this is no longer tenable; it is more realistic, and fits in more acceptably with currently held concepts of integration of cerebral structure and function, to recognize that several neurotransmitters are affected collectively in any one clinical disorder.

PSYCHOPHYSIOLOGICAL BASIS OF EMOTIONAL EXPERIENCE[18,33,34]

Fundamental to any emotional experience is an appropriate cognitive state combined with a degree of arousal; this, necessarily, involves stimulation of the reticular formation in the brainstem, various thalamic nuclei and parts of the neocortex. The hypothalamus, too, is involved in activating the accompanying visceral changes; it regulates both the endocrine system and the autonomic nervous system and is, itself, powerfully influenced by the limbic system which, in turn, has an important input from the neocortex, particularly the frontal lobe. The limbic system also has an important input to the reticular activating system and is, therefore, a route by which cortical stimulation can create arousal.

Hence, emotion depends on the coordination of several systems – the cortical system (to initiate an appropriate cognitive state), the limbic structures (to activate the brainstem, thalamic activating centres and the hypothalamus), the hypothalamus (to activate endocrine and autonomic responses) and the brainstem and thalamic activating system (to stimulate cortical arousal).

EXPERIMENTAL OBSERVATIONS

Stimulation of many hypothalamic and other limbic centres, such as the septum, nucleus accumbens, hypothalamic ventromedial nuclei and the median forebrain bundle *via* an electrode, is able to produce pleasurable experience. An animal with an indwelling electrode soon learns to effectively control its own stimulation so as to produce 'perpetual reward', with accompanying docility and apparent tranquillity. Should stimulation be directed to the fornical nucleus of the hypothalamus and mesencephalic grey matter, however, then the consequence is very different; pain and emotional displeasure occur. In this context, it is firmly established that stimulation of the hippocampus and amygdala in man produces a somewhat unpleasant experience. A 'rage response' ensues from stimulation of the perifornical nucleus, but more rostral stimulation merely causes fear and anxiety.

Sleep and wakefulness, too, is promoted by activating other areas in the vicinity, acting by way of hypothalamic influence over the reticular system. Stimulation dorsal to the mammillary bodies produces alertness, excitement and excessive sympathetic activity; whereas somnolence or sleep results if the electrode lies in certain parts of the septum, anterior hypothalamus or thalamic reticular nuclei. The 'fight, flight and fright response', that typifies sympathetic activity, is universally familiar. Regulation of autonomic activity by way of hypothalamic nuclei has already been alluded to. Memory with its complex NA and ACh involvements has also been the subject of much experimentation.

4
Neurotransmitters and psychiatric disorders

The psychiatric disorders included in this section will be dealt with primarily from the angle of their neurotransmitter involvements; any other biochemical, physiological, clinical and genetic abnormalities will either not be included or only cursorily documented.

SCHIZOPHRENIA[30,35–38]

In developed countries schizophrenia occurs in approximately one per cent of the adult population at some point during their lives. It comprises a group of psychoses with either 'positive' or 'negative' symptoms. Positive symptoms consist of hallucinations, delusions and disorders of thought; negative symptoms include emotional flattening, lack of volition and a decrease in motor activity. The two syndromes alluded to above are called type-1 and type-2 schizophrenia, respectively; it is the former which is likely to be associated with hyperactivity of the dopaminergic system centrally.

A number of biochemical abnormalities have been identified and, in consequence, several neurotransmitter-based hypotheses have been advanced over recent years; the most popular one has been 'the dopamine hypothesis', one variant of which states that there is overactivity of the mesolimbic DA pathways at the level of the D_2 receptor. It is, therefore, important to recognize that it is not only the actual neurotransmitters but also the precise cerebral location of activity of each that are essential to know when establishing the nature of such a disorder. The undoubted genetic association in this case can be regarded as strong evidence for the presence of some metabolic defect.

In addition to the three hypotheses which are briefly presented here, and which attempt to draw together the neurochemical observations in schizophrenia, one should add that some abnormalities of cortical neuropeptides are documented. The latter include changes in the levels of somatostatin, substance P, CCK and VIP found in association with negative symptom defect states in the temporal area of the brain (i.e. the hippocampus, amygdala and neocortex), in particular.

Dopamine involvement

Administration of amphetamines and amphetamine-like drugs increases DA release in normal volunteers; in parallel with this enhanced dopaminergic neurotransmission, there is intensification of the positive symptoms of the disorder in a patient with schizophrenia. On the other hand, neuroleptic drugs effectively cause DA receptor blockade by occupying the DA receptors, thus blocking the effect of DA on post-synaptic structures. In parallel with this reduced dopaminergic neurotransmission there is amelioration of the positive symptoms of schizophrenia. To be more precise, the antipsychotic potency of such drugs parallels blocking activity involving the D_2, rather than the D_1, receptor. The highly selective D_2 receptor antagonists, sulpiride and remoxipride (both being substituted benzamide compounds), are just two of the antipsychotic drugs used in the treatment of schizophrenia. Clozapine, too, sometimes successful in the therapy of severe and intractable schizophrenia, causes blockade of the D_2 receptors – but is of weaker action than other neuroleptic agents in not causing elevation of serum prolactin (PRL). However, successful therapeutic effect may be based on antagonism of both D_2 and $5HT_2$ receptors. The earlier finding of an elevated number of D_2 binding sites in postmortem brain tissue of patients with schizophrenia might be simply a compensatory response to the effect of antipsychotic drugs over a long period of time, rather than being due to the disease itself. Moreover, the findings are not fully supported by recent studies of positron emission tomography (PET) scanning in patients who had not received such drug treatment.

However, there are other observations which do not seem to support 'the dopamine hypothesis' entirely. One is that the beneficial therapeutic response to DA antagonist compounds, leading to dopaminergic blockade, can take at least two weeks to emerge. Also, schizophrenia can co-exist with Parkinson's disease. Moreover, the 'core' symptoms of schizophrenia do not always respond successfully to treatment with antipsychotic drugs.

Catecholamine involvement

Catecholamines undergo methylation as part of the normal metabolic processes. It is of great interest in this context, that mescaline and other psychotic agents chemically resemble the methylated derivatives of the catecholamines. Moreover, in schizophrenic patients, the enzymes involved in one-carbon (methyl) metabolism are reduced. The suggestion, therefore, is that some of the oxidation products of adrenaline may be psychomimetic or hallucinogenic, thus producing behavioural changes. Hence, should the amine supply be increased, or its catabolism prevented by inhibition of MAO, then amines could, theoretically, be transmethylated to hallucinogens; this is sometimes referred to as the 'transmethylation hypothesis'.

Glutamate involvement

Glutamic and aspartic acids are both excitatory neurotransmitters in the CNS. In a study on schizophrenic patients the cerebrospinal fluid (CSF) glutamate concentration was found to be half that of control subjects, whereas there was no such difference in the serum glutamate values; the suggestion was that this was because of some dysfunction of the glutamatergic neurones. Of considerable interest is the effect of D-amphetamine in animals – which leads to a rise of dopaminergic function in the frontal cortex, striatum and hippocampus, leading to increased concentrations of glutamate levels in the CSF. Phencyclidine, an NMDA (*N*-methyl-D-aspartate) antagonist, can mimic the symptoms of paranoid schizophrenia when given to a normal individual; if given to a schizophrenic patient, however, it can exacerbate the symptoms. The glutamate receptors are concentrated in the area of the hippocampus; also, glutamate receptor densities are reduced in the temporal regions in postmortem brain tissue.

DEPRESSION[30,38,39]

Depression, characterized by a pathological lowering of mood of more severe degree and of longer duration than those swings which occur in normal circumstances, is traditionally regarded as either reactive to life-events or endogenous; stress may be a precipitating factor in either case. In equilibrium with the change of mood there are biological accompaniments such as disturbance of sleep pattern with a tendency to early morning wakening, loss of appetite, loss of weight and a lessening or loss of libido.

Many neurochemical findings are coming to light implicating a biological basis for the 'functional disorders' (depression and anxiety), at least for certain subtypes. Abnormalities of monoamine function have been recognized in depression for many years, not only involving NA but also DA and 5HT. Other evidence along these lines will now be briefly documented. Studies of cation transport across red cell membranes suggest that there is an abnormality of cell membrane function in manic depressive illness.

Noradrenaline involvement

Amphetamine administration has long been known to elevate mood; this is known to be accompanied by increased activity of noradrenergic and dopaminergic neurones. However, the introduction of reserpine, used in the therapy of hypertension in the early 1950s, revealed that some patients so treated developed depression; it was found that the drug depleted neuronal stores of monoamines. Hence, it was surmised that those patients suffering from endogenous depression might, perhaps, possess inability to naturally produce sufficient monoamines for neuronal transmission. In keeping with the 'noradrenergic hypothesis' was the later observation that antidepressant drugs were observed to potentiate monoamine neurotransmission, increasing either NA or 5HT at aminergic synapses. Moreover, tricyclic antidepressants were found to inhibit the re-uptake mechanisms for NA and 5HT, thereby increasing synaptic concentrations of these amines; monoamine oxidase inhibitor (MAOI) drugs were found to do likewise. In excess of one hundred drugs, many of them structurally different from tricyclic compounds and MAOIs, have now been used in the treatment of depression, each one of which produces an increased amount of available NA and/or 5HT at the synaptic cleft.

Depression may be a feature in up to fifty per cent of patients with neurodegenerative disorders such as Parkinson's disease and Alzheimer's disease. The neuronal loss in the locus coeruleus, typical of Alzheimer's disease, is greatest in those patients who have depression and they also have lower NA levels than do those who lack depressive features. Approximately fifty per cent of patients with Alzheimer's disease have less NA than normal in the majority of cortical and subcortical areas of the brain that have been examined to date.

All these facts seem, at first reading, to fit neatly into this hypothesis; however, from later findings it becomes clear that some re-appraisal and modifications are necessary. The increased levels of monoamine transmitters at the synapses, although quickly produced in response to antidepressant therapy, are in contrast with the much slower clinical recovery of the patient from depression, which takes about two weeks to begin and which may only be maximal several weeks later. Moreover, should acute depletion of either NA and/or 5HT occur experimentally in a normal individual then depression does not, in the short-term, occur. Not seemingly in keeping with the hypothesis, too, is the cerebral resistance generated in response to the pharmacological changes induced by antidepressant compounds. These counteractive changes comprise reduction in the number of post-synaptic β-receptors, together with a lowered firing rate of noradrenergic neurones.

Serotonin involvement

Dysfunction of 5HT metabolism, as shown by decreased concentrations of the metabolite 5HIAA in CSF, was found to be linked with depression; nevertheless, it was not a feature in all patients with depression – hence, a subgroup entitled 'serotonin depression' was proposed. A reduction in the number of 5HT-containing neurones in the median raphe in Parkinson's disease, Alzheimer's disease and, possibly, also in the elderly, is associated with the development of depression.

Acetylcholine involvement

Many antidepressant drugs have an anticholinergic effect, which lends support to the suggestion that in depression there might be some centrally increased cholinergic tone. In this context, anticholinergic compounds are in themselves mood-elevating, whereas cholinomimetics can induce marked depression. Nevertheless, there is no evidence at postmortem examination for cholinergic abnormality in such patients.

Dopamine involvement

Low levels of the DA metabolite HVA are found in the CSF in patients with depression. In addition, DA agonists produce a therapeutic response in depression.

MANIA/HYPOMANIA[38,40]

Mania or hypomania comprises one phase of manic depressive psychosis (bipolar manic depression). Clinical presentation may take the form of irritability, restlessness, elation, euphoria, increased talkativeness at rapid rate, increased energy, increased appetite for food, overactivity, hostility, aggressiveness, delusions of grandeur, an inflated self-esteem, loss of insight, easy distractibility, a decreased need for sleep and social and sexual disinhibition. There may, in addition, be revealed 'flight of ideas' and a subjective feeling of 'racing of thoughts'. Furthermore, the patient may be found to be extravagantly spending money and to be becoming involved in financially unsound business schemes.

Reference has already been made to an abnormality of cation transport across red cell membranes in manic depressive illness.

Noradrenaline involvement

Functional overactivity of catecholamine neurotransmission (i.e. either excess of the amines themselves or hypersensitivity of their receptors) may be the fundamental difference between mania/hypomania and depression (where there is receptor insensitivity and depletion of amines, together with a reduction in their synthesis and storage). Drugs that enhance catecholamine neurotransmission can lead to the onset of mania (e.g. MAOIs, tricyclic antidepressant compounds, levodopa, etc.), whereas lithium carbonate leads to destruction of these amines at the nerve endings, thereby causing less to be released; hence, there may also be reduced sensitivity of postsynaptic receptor sites. There is evidence for an increase in urinary and CSF levels of NA and its metabolite 3-methoxy-4-hydroxyphenylethylene glycol (MOPEG) in manic patients; there is, too, increased activity of the enzyme DBH (involved in the conversion of DA to NA) in contrast to the decrease which is found in depression.

Acetylcholine involvement

A decrease in central cholinergic tone is implicated in mania/hypomania, as opposed to the presumed increase of such activity in depression. In this context, it is postulated that balance between the adrenergic and cholinergic systems accounts for mood stability; imbalance between the two systems would, therefore, lead to mood instability.

ANXIETY[30,38,41,42]

The clinical expression of anxiety, in its different forms, includes both psychological and biological symptoms. From the psychological aspect there may be fear, irritability and restlessness, together with excessive sensitivity to noise, impairment of concentration and sleep disturbance. The biological accompaniments of anxiety comprise the consequences of autonomic overactivity, skeletal muscle tension and the effects of hyperventilation. Autonomic overactivity leads to palpitations and sweating, dryness of the mouth, diarrhoea, frequency of micturition and, sexually, to impotence or frigidity; muscular tension can cause headache and aching lower down – in the neck and in the back. Hyperventilation can cause the patient to feel dizzy or faint, with paraesthesiae and palpitations. Similar symptoms, presenting suddenly, in marked degree and perhaps of unexpected onset, are referred to as 'panic attacks'; symptoms comprise combinations of the following – palpitations, breathlessness, sweating, trembling, a feeling of dizziness or faintness, paraesthesiae or numbness, flushing and nausea, together with depersonalization and a fear of impending death.

Evidence is accumulating for there being a biological basis to anxiety, as there also is for the other 'functional disorder', i.e. depression; the biochemical observations revealed in anxiety now follow.

Noradrenaline involvement

The physiological release of catecholamines occurs in the 'fight, flight and fright' response to a stressful situation. The turnover of NA is reduced in response to benzodiazepine compounds. Also, the α_2 adrenergic receptor antagonist clonidine is anxiolytic.

GABA involvement

GABA is the major of two inhibitory amino acid neurotransmitters, the other being glycine. The $GABA_A$ receptor possesses a chloride channel complex; it has at least four separate binding sites, one of which binds benzodiazepine drugs, anxiolytic compounds and β-carbolines. Benzodiazepine binding occurs to a high degree in the cerebral cortex and amygdala; in some way it seems to unmask GABA receptors in many areas of the brain, thereby permitting enhanced GABA binding, with the consequence of optimal GABA-ergic neuronal activity, i.e. inhibitory in function.

Endogenous anxiolytics and, perhaps, anxiogenic molecules, too, may both exist *in vivo*; it is possible that a 104 long amino acid peptide, called diazepam-binding-inhibitor, which possesses the ability to markedly reduce the duration of opening of ion channels, is a candidate.

Serotonin involvement

Buspirone and ipsapirone are anxiolytic drugs which possess antagonist action by selectively binding to the autoreceptor subtype $5HT_{1A}$; these receptors are located on cell bodies of the serotoninergic neurones in the brainstem.

ALZHEIMER'S DISEASE[30,43-45]

Alzheimer's disease is characterized by the onset in middle age of a slowly progressive dementia; there is loss of memory for past events, inability to lay down new memories and impairment of intellect – all leading to a lessened capacity for dealing with the tasks and problems of daily living. It is the commonest cause of both presenile and senile dementia. Alzheimer's disease is not the non-specific degenerative disorder of the CNS that it was once thought to be, as neurochemical studies on postmortem material now reveal the degeneration to be selective for certain neuronal populations in the subcortical and cortical areas; other cell populations seem to be unaffected. Senile plaques and neurofibrillary tangles are the characteristic histological feature, found throughout the cerebral cortex and especially in certain regions of the limbic system (the amygdala and hippocampus), perhaps accounting for the memory loss so typical of the early phase of the disease. There is reduction of ACh, NA, 5HT and somatostatin in the subcortical areas in Alzheimer's disease. Superimposed upon the mental retardation of Down syndrome, in all who are over 40 years of age, is dementia – with a pathology identical to that seen in patients with Alzheimer's disease.

Acetylcholine involvement

The activity of CAT, the enzyme involved in ACh synthesis, is markedly decreased in Alzheimer's disease. This decrease does not occur in all areas of the brain, but does so particularly in the hippocampus and amygdala, which are some of the main sites where senile plaques and neurofibrillary tangles accumulate. The loss of such cortical cholinergic activity correlates well with the degree of dementia in patients with this disease. In keeping with these findings, anticholinergic drugs are found to disrupt memory in normal individuals; on the other hand, cholinergic drugs, such as anticholinesterases (e.g. tetrahydroaminoacridine) and muscarinic or nicotinic acid agonists (e.g. bethanechol or nicotine) do not seem to help the memories of all patients – and then, at best, only partially in those who do respond. A further finding is that nerve growth factor (NGF) is now known to be involved in the maintenance of cholinergic neurones in the forebrain; also, nicotine, a cholinomimetic compound, is able to stimulate dopaminergic neurones *via* their nicotinic receptors – thus, seemingly, to provide smokers with some protection against degeneration of the dopaminergic neurones. The forebrain cholinergic system degenerates not only in Alzheimer's disease, but also in alcohol-induced dementia, Pick's disease, Lewy body dementia, progressive supranuclear palsy and in Parkinson's disease.

Glutamate involvement

The cortical areas of the brain that are mainly affected in Alzheimer's disease are probably innervated by glutamate fibres. Of special note is the fact that excitatory amino acids are able, *in vitro*, to induce the formation of neurofibrillary tangles; however, they do also occur in some other disorders of the CNS.

Serotonin involvement

In Alzheimer's disease there is a reduction of both 5HT and its receptor protein in the temporal lobe of the brain, as revealed from studies on autopsy and biopsy material. The loss of 5HT is, however, less than in Parkinson's disease and it would be unlikely, therefore, that the severe memory loss of Alzheimer's disease could be accounted for on this basis alone, although in Parkinson's disease there is an important difference in that the $5HT_2$ receptor is not decreased. Of interest in this context, but not necessarily related, is the bradyphrenia (characterized by difficulty in concentration, slowing of thought processes and inability to associate ideas) of Parkinson's disease where 5HT is low in most of the cortical regions. In the Lewy body type of senile dementia it is common for visual hallucinations to occur, and it is of great interest that in the temporal lobe the serotoninergic activity is higher (as shown by the definitely raised serotoninergic:cholinergic ratio) in those patients who suffer from hallucinations compared with those who do not.

Noradrenaline involvement

It is in those patients with Alzheimer's disease who also have depression that there is not only greatest reduction in the number of neurones within the locus coeruleus but also a markedly reduced NA content.

Neuropeptide involvement

There is associated reduction in cortical somatostatin and CRF. Loss of the somatostatin content of neurones in the temporal cortex develops early in the condition.

5
Neuroendocrinological aspects of psychiatric disorders

Following an introduction to hormonal control by way of neurotransmitter compounds, come sections on schizophrenia, puerperal psychosis, depression, mania/hypomania and stress.

NEUROTRANSMITTERS AND HORMONES[40]

A neurotransmitter secreted by one neurone not only determines the response of other neurones with which it synapses (causing stimulation or inhibition accordingly) but also influences hormonal secretions should it project to the hypothalamus and pituitary gland. 5HT, DA, NA and ACh have all been shown to possess important control over the neuroendocrine system.

5HT-secreting neurones in the hypothalamus influence the release of various pituitary hormones, as assessed by their serum/plasma levels. In turn, such levels can be regarded as a measure of neurotransmission activity in the neuroendocrine pathways involved. Stimulation of 5HT-secreting neurones causes inhibition of the pituitary gonadotrophins, i.e. luteinizing hormone (LH) and follicle-stimulating hormone (FSH), but increases the release of adrenocorticotrophic hormone (ACTH), GH and PRL. In the pineal gland, large amounts of 5HT are synthesized within the pinealocytes, serving as precursor of melatonin (5-methoxy-N-acetyltryptamine) formation. Both 5HT and melatonin have a marked circadian variation, with maximal pineal melatonin production occurring during the dark phase of the photoperiod in all animals. In fact, melatonin is probably the coordinator of biological rhythms in the human, as it is in many animals. Exposure to bright light not only suppresses melatonin secretion but also has been shown to modify seasonal mood variation in those subjects who suffer from seasonal affective disorder (SAD) – with its accompanying depression of mood during the darker winter months[46–48].

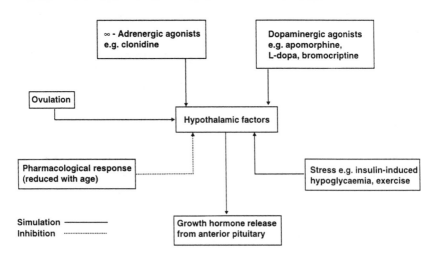

Figure 17 Neurotransmitter involvement in hormonal control. (Reproduced with permission from Mander, A.J. and Goodwin, G.M. (1990) Neuroendocrinology of psychiatric disorders. *Hospital Update*, March, 211–17)

GH is under the neurotransmitter control of 5HT, DA, NA, ACh and opioid peptides. It may be that 5HT acts as the final common pathway through which other neurotransmitters act. Stimulation of DA receptors, by administration of apomorphine (a DA agonist) or L-DOPA, evokes GH secretion in the normal individual, producing elevation of serum GH. This effect is blocked by haloperidol (a DA receptor antagonist) but not by domperidone (which is not able to cross the blood–brain barrier). It is likely, therefore, that a hypothalamic site, rather than a pituitary one, is the level at which GH is controlled. Stimulation of DA receptors, however, leads to inhibition of the excessive amounts of GH secreted in patients with acromegaly (Figure 17).

PRL secretion is controlled by DA at physiological level; it is also influenced by DA agonists and antagonists pharmacologically. Suppression of PRL is caused by tonic dopaminergic activity. DA agonists, therefore, enhance suppression, whereas both DA antagonists and inhibitors of DA synthesis remove the inhibitory effect of DA, thereby liberating increased amounts of hormone into the blood. Bromocriptine (a DA receptor agonist) is used therapeutically to suppress PRL secretion by pituitary adenomas. Another DA agonist, apomorphine, also suppresses PRL unless the level is very high to begin with. This latter effect is blocked by both haloperidol and domperidone. However, as domperidone does not cross the blood–brain barrier this indicates that the mechanism of action is by way of a direct action on the DA receptors in the pituitary gland.

SCHIZOPHRENIA[40]

In patients with acute schizophrenia and in those with positive symptoms, administration of apomorphine produces an enhanced serum GH response. However, in patients with chronic schizophrenia and in those with negative symptoms, a blunted response occurs. It may be that reduction in the sensitivity of receptors in those receiving chronic neuroleptic therapy partly explains the blunting of the GH response; age is probably an additional factor. In keeping with this suggestion is the finding that the maximum blunting is seen in those patients who have been receiving therapy for the longest period of time. Hyperkinetic involuntary movements of the face and neck (tardive dyskinesia), as a complication of drug therapy, is seen with highest frequency in this group of patients – and they also have a high incidence of blunted GH response to apomorphine provocation. When a single intravenous dose of haloperidol is given to a schizophrenic patient it causes less PRL to be released than is the case for normal controls.

PUERPERAL PSYCHOSIS[49-52]

In the first four weeks postpartum there is a 20-times higher incidence of psychotic illness than in the two years prior to this event. There is, at this time, a rapid fall of circulating oestradiol and progesterone, both of which (unlike many other hormones) have direct access to the brain structures. Monoaminergic and dopaminergic neurotransmitter systems are modulated by oestrogens; in consequence, it has been suggested that puerperal psychosis is precipitated by the rapid withdrawal of oestrogens at this time.

The response of the D_2 receptors in the hypothalamus (and other sites) to apomorphine has been assessed by studying the secretion of GH which follows. In one study, involving women with a past history of bipolar or schizoaffective psychosis, the result of giving 0.005 mg/kg of apomorphine hydrochloride subcutaneously on the fourth day postpartum was that the serum GH response was greater in those women who subsequently had recurrence of their psychotic disorder (in five cases it was a bipolar illness, in one case it was schizomanic and in two others the diagnosis was of a major depressive illness). The implication is that there is at this time an increased sensitivity of the DA receptors not only in the hypothalamus but also at the other sites.

DEPRESSION[40,53]

In depression there is hypothalamic–pituitary–adrenal axis 'overdrive' with early 'escape' from the serum cortisol suppression normally produced by a single dose of dexamethasone in the dexamethasone suppression test (DST). In addition, there is blunting of the serum thyroid-stimulating hormone (TSH) response to TRH. The true positive rate for these two tests is 44% and at least 20–30%, respectively; if both tests are performed in patients with 'endogenous' depression then 67% are abnormal on one or both tests. There is also blunting of the serum GH response to stimulation by precursors of 5HT (i.e. tryptophan and 5HTP). The serum PRL response mediated by 5HT is also reduced in depression; this is not, however, on account of an abnormality of PRL function as there is a normal PRL secretory response to the DA antagonist, metoclopramide – hence, the decreased levels are most likely to be accounted for by a functional deficit in 5HT neurotransmission.

Dexamethasone suppression test (DST) for depression[54]

The normal response of serum cortisol suppression, following a standard dose of dexamethasone given orally, is absent in approximately 50% of patients suffering from affective disorders with a significant element of endogenous depression; this is due to failure of negative feedback to suppress limbic system activity[54,55]. Prior to performing this test on either in-patients or out-patients, there should be no treatment with glucocorticoid drugs (including topical preparations) for several weeks; mineralocorticoids do not interfere with the test. Blood is collected for assay of serum cortisol at 09.00 h and 16.00 h on the first day. On the same evening at 23.00 h, dexamethasone (1.0 mg) is given orally. A further blood test is taken at 09.00 h and 16.00 h on the following day.

In a normal individual the baseline 09.00 h serum cortisol value on the first day should be within the reference range (140–460 nmol/l). There is marked suppression of the 09.00 h serum cortisol value on the second day (i.e. 10 h after the dexamethasone dose); this remains low at 16.00 h (<180 nmol/l) and persisting for a total period of 24 h.

A significant proportion (44%) of patients with depression (in whom there is loss of the normal diurnal variation in serum cortisol levels) show early 'escape' from the suppression of serum cortisol normally seen at 16.00 h on the second day, as evidenced by a concentration of >180 nmol/l, or of >50% of the value found at 16.00 h on the first day. However, many patients with depression fail to show this early 'escape' by exhibiting a low serum cortisol concentration at this time, i.e. a false negative result. A recent study of patients with endogenous depression revealed the sensitivity (true positive rate) in the DST to be 44%; the specificity (true negative rate) was >90% (when compared with normal controls) and 77% (when compared with patients suffering from other psychiatric disorders).

Low serum cortisol concentrations may also be found in individuals with organic hypofunction of the adrenal cortex or anterior pituitary gland, but these patients would show low levels in the baseline sample, too. Marked hepatic microsomal P_{450} enzyme induction, as caused by a number of drugs (e.g. phenobarbitone, other anticonvulsants and benzodiazepines) may interfere with the test by causing dexamethasone to be eliminated unduly rapidly, thereby causing inadequate suppression of serum cortisol. Some patients with other disorders, including anorexia nervosa without obvious depression, weight loss from other causes, schizophrenia, mania, obsessive–compulsive neurosis and patients with dementia associated with enlarged cerebral ventricles, show false positive responses, i.e. they, too, display 'escape' from suppression. Less than 10% of normal subjects also show a positive response. The test is negative in patients with pure anxiety states, but it must be remembered that this and other psychiatric disorders may be associated with an element of depression, in which case the test could be positive. A repeat test following treatment for the depression, which remains positive, suggests a poor prognosis.

If the 09.00 h blood sample taken on the second day shows a low serum cortisol concentration as compared with a normal baseline value on the first day, this confirms compliance with the taking of an adequate dose of dexamethasone. This knowledge is important when assessing depressed patients exhibiting early 'escape' (i.e. by finding normal serum cortisol levels at 16.00 h on the second day). Some authorities recommend measurement of serum dexamethasone concentrations as a further check on compliance, in addition to assaying serum cortisol. Dexamethasone does not interfere with the measurement of serum cortisol. There is continuing discussion and some difference of opinion in the literature concerning the value of this test, and some authorities would advocate a prolonged suppression test, in which there would be increased significance of a positive result[54].

Thyrotrophin-releasing hormone (TRH) stimulation test

Thyrotrophin-releasing hormone (TRH) stimulates the synthesis and release of thyroid-stimulating hormone (TSH) and PRL from the anterior pituitary gland. In hyperthyroidism administration of exogenous TRH is characterized by impaired release of TSH, whereas in primary hypothyroidism there is exaggerated release; in both instances there is altered target organ feedback. In hypothalamic disorders the TSH response is delayed on account of time being required for its synthesis within the pituitary gland. Ideally, the patient should fast overnight and during the test, and be at rest. Smoking is not permitted. The best time for the test is early in the morning. Venous blood is collected, following which an injection of TRH (200 µg) is given intravenously as a bolus. Further blood samples are collected at 20 and 60 min.

In a normal individual the baseline level of serum TSH should be <7 mIU/l, with a significant rise of >2 mIU/l (but with peak <25 mIU/l) at 20 min in response to TRH, and with return towards the baseline value at 60 min. In this test a flat or nearly flat response (i.e. a serum TSH rise of <2 mIU/l) with a low baseline level occurs in hyperthyroidism, including the early stages of the disease. Early primary hypothyroidism displays a high baseline level together with an exaggerated response at 20 min. It is important to exclude hypofunction of the anterior pituitary gland whenever there is an impaired response; this may also occur in acromegaly, Cushing's syndrome, after adrenocortical steroid therapy and following previous thyroid therapy. A delayed peak occurs in hypothalamic disease, with the 60 min sample showing a higher level than the 20 min sample. An exaggerated response is seen in pregnancy and in patients receiving oral contraceptives. In cases of reduced end-organ sensitivity to circulating thyroid hormones, there may be an elevated response in this test. Normal elderly subjects show a smaller rise of serum TSH, but always >2 mIU/l. In patients with chronic renal failure or liver disease the serum TSH response to TRH is prolonged but delayed. Occasionally, apparently healthy subjects fail to respond. Drugs which modify the TSH response include antithyroid compounds, L-DOPA, phenothiazines, metoclopramide, bromocriptine, salicylates and theophylline; thyroxine (T_4) and tri-iodothyronine (T_3) administration will affect the response.

In some patients with depression there is blunting of the TSH response, with a return to normal values following clinical recovery. The sensitivity (true positive rate) of the test in depression is at least 20–30% and the specificity (true negative rate) is >95% when compared with normal controls. Those patients with severe endogenous depression, perhaps with psychotic features, are more likely to have an abnormal response in this test. Possible causes of the blunted response include an increased inhibitory feedback from circulating thyroid hormones, pituitary gland dysfunction secondary to weight loss (possibly more likely in women) and chronic biological disorders of non-endocrine origin[56].

Clonidine stimulation test[57]

Clonidine stimulates GH release from the anterior pituitary gland, causing elevation of serum GH levels, thus serving as a test of anterior pituitary function. The patient should be investigated under 'basal conditions', except that there is no restriction of water intake. Clonidine is administered orally as 25 µg Dixarit tablets (Boehringer Ingelheim Ltd.) in a dose of 0.15 mg/m² of body surface area and rounded up to the nearest whole number of tablets. Blood pressure is monitored at 30 min intervals throughout the test and for a further 3 h afterwards. Venous blood is collected at 0, 30, 60, 90, 120, 150 and 180 min. An intravenous catheter inserted 30 min prior to collection of the first blood sample should be used. A note of caution should be made in that drowsiness and hypotension may be side effects for up to 3 h, and continuing bed rest is, therefore, essential. The normal response is for the serum GH to rise steeply from <10 mIU/l to >20 mIU/l at 60–120 min after clonidine administration. An inadequate response is seen in GH deficiency, either as an isolated state or as part of panhypopituitarism. A poor response may also occur in primary hypothyroidism. In some children, social deprivation also leads to an inadequate response, as also is the case in endogenous depressive illness in adults[57].

MANIA/HYPOMANIA[38,40]

In acute mania, the highest serum levels of the stress hormones cortisol and PRL are found in the most psychotic patients; in young males there is also elevation of serum LH.

STRESS[58–61]

Psychological stress is characterized mentally by changes in cognitive processes, affect and behaviour, but there is also the accompanying impact on physiological mechanisms. There will be variability of response between individuals and there may even be changes in the same person at different times. Also influential are genetic inheritance, the past experience of an individual and the current state of health.

The psychological response to a stressful situation is closely integrated with a change of motor activity, stimulation of the autonomic nervous system and an endocrine system response.

The autonomic nervous system comprises sympathetic and parasympathetic components. Stimulation of the sympathetic nervous system leads to many physiological changes including an increase in heart rate and myocardial contractility, vasodilatation in skeletal muscle and constriction of blood vessels in the skin and gastrointestinal tract. There is, in consequence, a deviation in blood supply to skeletal muscle, the heart and the brain (i.e. the organs required in the 'fight, flight and fright' response), at the same time as temporarily conserving the blood supply to organs of lesser need (e.g. the skin and gastrointestinal tract). Stimulation of the parasympathetic nervous system may not only cause emotional fainting (involving the vagus nerve), but also can provoke the onset of hyperventilation, which can itself contribute to states of panic.

The neuroendocrine response to stress involves not only changes in the hypothalamic–pituitary–adrenocortical axis (the most important being the increased ACTH secretion, which secondarily determines the adrenocortical response) but also alteration in the sympathetic–adrenomedullary system (causing catecholamines to be released from the adrenal medulla).

Psychological stress also promotes secretion of other hormones (e.g. GH, PRL, insulin and testosterone). In addition, there is involvement of the opioid peptide system. Opioid secretion may serve as a mechanism for preventing too much activation of the sympathetic nervous system at times of stress, thereby limiting catecholamine secretion.

6

Psychiatric disorders and clinical chemistry

The information supplied in previous chapters of this book provides some understanding of the anatomical and physiological basis of the equilibrium between the mind and its chemistry. Many more aspects other than neurotransmitters themselves could have been discussed; neurotransmitters are influenced by yet other chemical processes, the details of which are outside the main theme of this account – but which, nevertheless, must be referred to, however briefly. Oestrogens, for instance, are known to modulate CNS monoaminergic and dopaminergic neurotransmitter systems, melatonin (physiologically involved in the light–dark cycle) is integrally involved in the generation of SAD – and increase of CNS serotoninergic activity is effective not only in suppressing dietary carbohydrate intake but also in producing a favourable clinical response in SAD[48].

ENDOCRINE DISORDERS[62–65]

It is well known that emotional changes occur at certain times of life with greater frequency. Many of these are related to functional changes in the endocrine system. Puberty, menstruation, pregnancy and the menopause are physiological stresses which might underlie such behavioural changes. There should be no surprise that endocrine disturbances of a pathological nature are also associated with mood changes (e.g. Addison's disease and depression, hypothyroidism and depression, thyrotoxicosis and hyperdynamism, exposure to anabolic steroid drugs and aggression, etc.). In this context it is important to note that T_4 is so fundamental to the proper development of cerebral structure and function, that without it (i.e. cretinism) there can be no normal intellectual development. Clearly, there is a close relationship between endocrinology and psychiatry, but reference must also be made to the endocrine consequences of some primary emotional disturbances (e.g. the missed menstrual period at a time of anxiety, the increased sympathetic activity with rise of the associated circulating hormones at times of anger and tension, etc.).

Hyperthyroidism[62,65–67]

Clinical aspects

The typical mood changes comprise irritability, nervousness and restlessness, together with increased dynamism and tremulousness. Emotional lability may occur and depression is sometimes a feature; apathetic thyrotoxicosis is a rare presentation. Thyrotoxic crisis (with its accompanying delirium), although very rare, constitutes a grave emergency; it can be precipitated by acute infection, surgery for thyrotoxicosis and may even follow soon after severe stress, injury or an emotional crisis. The difficulty is being certain that the initial emotional reaction did not occur on the basis of already present but unrecognized overactivity of the thyroid gland. Affective and schizophrenic psychoses sometimes occur, with mania being more likely than depression.

The cause of the mood changes is probably increased circulating T_4; cerebral catecholamines are also intimately involved. The pronounced adrenergic manifestations of thyrotoxicosis include sweating, tremor and tachycardia; all these can be relieved by therapy with propanolol.

Biochemical basis

Maintenance of the Na^+/K^+-ATPase pump requires much of the total energy utilized by a cell, together with O_2 and thyroid hormone. Excessive amounts of the latter lead to increased oxidative phosphorylation, thereby leading to elevated O_2 consumption with associated enhanced ATP utilization. Thyroid hormone also produces a positive nitrogen balance, by increasing protein synthesis. It also enhances transcription of the GH gene (leading to more GH production) and is involved in developmental processes (e.g. intrauterine and neonatal thyroid development, in the absence of which cretinism results).

Hypothyroidism[62,65–67]

Clinical aspects

The usual insidiously slow onset is a prime reason for the diagnosis being so often missed in the early stages. There is both mental and physical slowing, with progressive difficulty in understanding, loss of initative, onset of lethargy and development of apathy. Initially, the patient may have insight to the changes taking place, at the time when forgetfulness and failure to recall events is just beginning. Depression, dementia and organic psychoses can all occur, these usually being of gradual onset. Intellectual impairment is reversible if the condition is not left untreated for too long; depression, too, is often relieved by thyroid replacement therapy. 'Myxoedema madness' could include dementia, depression or schizophrenia. Myxoedema coma is the end-stage of the condition if left untreated, although precipitating factors include infection, injury, exposure to cold and administration of CNS depressants. Hypothyroidism in children may present as poor school performance, and in the first weeks of life cretinism can be the basis of impaired mental development.

Biochemical basis

Deficiency of circulating T_4 and increased TSH occur, together with decreased cerebral blood flow (caused by reduction in cardiac output), anaemia and relative cerebral hypoxia. Dilutional hyponatraemia with cerebral hydraemia may contribute to mental symptoms – and so, too, may CO_2 retention in myxoedema pre-coma/coma. In early life, T_4 is necessary for brain development.

CASE 1

Clinical history

A 20-year-old male student who had shown no outward indication of having been unwell, in the sense that there had been no evident change of personality, was found on 01.07.85 (after a week-end) hanging in his room in the residency of the university where he had been studying. There were no suspicious circumstances.

According to his general practitioner he was known to possess a manic–depressive character; this had first been recognized by his parents when he was just 9 years of age. Over the years his behaviour was episodically irrational and manic; there were 'highs' and 'lows', the spasms of enthusiasm coinciding with 'highs'. During recent months he had been consuming alcohol in large amounts. He had also just undergone his end-of-year examinations, together with all the pressures that they would normally entail.

He had entered the university one year previously, in September 1984, full of enthusiasm. However, over the year his enthusiasm had waned, and by Easter he was somewhat undecided as to whether to continue the course. He had said that, should he leave, he would simply find a job of some sort. Soon after this he had actually made a firm decision to resign and had decided it was time to inform the university authorities of his decision. He had already completed his examinations, but had not yet had the results. Over the few days prior to his death he had spent time at home with his parents. They had observed him to be more relaxed than was usual, not showing any of the signs of his more generally expressed difficult temperament, in which he resented any form of correction or advice. During these few days he had spoken more understandingly than for many years, and had been 'very lovable'. It was agreed, with his parents' full approval, that he should leave his studies. Accordingly, he went away cheerfully; his parents were expecting him to return in about 2 days time, either on the Sunday or Monday, and he called out 'I'll be back with my dirty washing'.

Laboratory investigations

At postmortem examination, which revealed no evidence of natural disease, tests were performed for alcohol, cannabis, cocaine and other drugs. Blood cannabis was very high at 176 µg/l, but alcohol, cocaine and other drugs were not detected.

Analysis and comments

In his room at the university residency were found small samples of cocaine and heroin, together with some cannabis – although there was no evidence that he had ever used the former two substances; they may well have been just 'collectors items'. A letter from the university authorities also came to light after his death, warning him that he would be dismissed if he continued failing to attend lectures. However, this would have been of no concern to him because by that time he had already decided not to continue the course. In addition, it emerged that his younger sister had been aware, over the last 2 years, of his interest in smoking cannabis. This was confirmed, too, by one of his friends. The death of this young man was a tremendous shock to his parents, family and friends. It was so unexpected and, seemingly, inexplicable – with there being no other known personal or social problems.

However, 5 years later, on 02.07.90, it was learned by chance that his younger sister, who by this time was the same age as he was at the time of his death, had been unwell for some months with increasing lethargy and irritability; she had also complained that her hair was falling out. Following a visit to the general practitioner she was referred to hospital where a diagnosis of hypothyroidism was made. She was commenced on thyroxine therapy. Shortly after this her father, who had not only become deaf over the last year but also had gained weight, was screened for hypothyroidism. He, too, was found to be positive and was started on thyroxine therapy.

Knowledge of the hereditary nature of autoimmune diseases must raise the distinct possibility, in retrospect, that this young man might have been developing subclinical hypothyroidism – with the features of depression and/or some other psychiatric instability preceding the more overt biological manifestations upon which the clinical diagnosis is usually based. The insidious onset of such depression could be the cause of a lowering of the threshold of response to other stresses. There can, of course, be no certainty that hypothyroidism was even present, or if it were present that it was in any way contributory to the situation. Nevertheless, it does seem important to bring the possibility to mind because, if it was true, then it could go a long way towards providing a more rational construction and understanding of the circumstances surrounding this suicide. It must, of course, remain conjecture as to whether cannabis itself might have played some part – if only in inducing the necessary state of mind prior to the final event. Moreover, the actual phase of mood of his manic–depressive character could have been a determining factor.

Cushing's syndrome[62,65]

Clinical aspects

There are several well-established causes of Cushing's syndrome, amongst which are: (i) excessive ACTH production by the pituitary gland (Cushing's disease) leading to bilateral adrenocortical hyperplasia, (ii) an adrenocortical adenoma or carcinoma, (iii) ACTH secretion by a bronchial carcinoma, (iv) steroid therapy in pharmacological doses (as opposed to the replacement doses required in Addison's disease) and (v) alcohol-induced Cushing's syndrome.

Psychiatric features are often found in Cushing's syndrome, depression being the commonest. Other symptoms sometimes seen include fatigue, emotional lability, irritability, agitation, restlessness and anxiety. Less commonly present are the more severe disorders of confusion, paranoia, frank schizophrenic psychosis and stupor. It is relatively uncommon, however, for any of the severe psychiatric features to accompany adrenal adenoma or carcinoma; it is in Cushing's disease that depression is so typical. Elevation of mood is often observed when steroids (in pharmacological doses) or ACTH therapy are given, some patients even becoming hypomanic when the dose is excessively high. The treatment of Cushing's syndrome usually leads to concomitant improvement of both biological and mental symptoms.

Biochemical basis

The aetiology of the mental symptoms may relate to electrolyte and H_2O distribution changes within the brain; there is, however, evidence in some patients of cerebral atrophy and ventricular enlargement. No doubt, an element of reactive depression is also involved on account of the embarrassment felt by the patients in view of their facial and other body changes. It is possible, too, that there is a close link in some way between the origin of both Cushing's disease and endogenous depression. Indeed, not only is there in endogenous depression an 'overdrive' of the hypothalamic–pituitary–adrenocortical axis (thus suggesting a link with the limbic system), but also there is a high incidence of factors predisposing to depression in patients with Cushing's disease.

Addison's disease[62,65]

Clinical aspects

Addison's disease is most often of autoimmune origin, but it can also be caused by infiltration of the adrenal cortex with tumour (e.g. carcinomatosis, or other tumour deposits), granuloma or tuberculosis; occasionally, there is bilateral haemorrhage into the glands. There is nearly always some mental involvement at initial presentation, the most typical features being apathy, lethargy, negativism and poverty of thought. Sometimes there is up to 2 years of psychiatric illness (e.g. depression) preceding the diagnosis. There can also be lack of drive and initiative, perhaps with rapid changes of mood, irritability, anxiety, restlessness, drowsiness and insomnia. More severe features, although less often seen, are paranoia and delusions.

Prior to an Addisonian crisis there may be exacerbation of certain mental feelings – such as apprehension, increasing irritability and even panic attacks. As the condition unfolds there is the onset of shock, with accompanying clouding of consciousness, delirium and stupor; at this point the clinical signs of shock are very apparent.

Biochemical basis

There is increased CRF and ACTH secretion in this disorder, accompanying the glucocorticoid deficiency; these factors could be the basis for neurotransmitter imbalance which, in turn, might influence β-adrenergic receptors and serotoninergic pathways. Electrolyte disturbances, found in the later stages of the disorder, may also contribute to the neuropsychiatric presentation.

CASE 2

Clinical history

A 27-year-old lady had had depression for just over 2 years. She would burst into tears for no apparent reason, felt apathetic, lacked motivation, felt that her mind had slowed down, was unable to work to her normal potential, was not able to concentrate properly and had impaired

---

memory. She lacked interest generally and in social communication. She had felt guilty about being ill and her inability to 'pull out of it'. There was no evidence of diurnal variation of mood and there was no insomnia. It was considered possible that she might have post-viral depression and treatment with amitriptyline was started. The depression began to 'lift' about 3 weeks later but she remained off work for a further 2 months. Nevertheless, since that time there had been intermittent depression, although this gradually became less intense with longer periods of normality in between the depressive episodes. She had been taking amitriptyline 50–125 mg nocte at different times over the 2-year period. She claimed that whenever she ceased taking the drug the depressive symptoms returned, and that if she took it in the daytime she suffered from excessive sedation.

It was established from her husband that she possessed a dependent personality. He said that a major problem was the dependency on both her mother and himself for even very trivial things, particularly noticeable on account of them having lived with her parents for nearly a year pending moving to their own new house which was nearing completion. He hoped that this move would lessen both the dependency and the depressive symptoms.

However, on 20.11 84, in addition to the depression of 2 years standing, the patient complained of loss of weight, and from that time onwards the illness progressively unfolded at a greater rate. She began to feel tired all day and there was general lack of energy. On 14.12.84 she was admitted to hospital complaining of lassitude, lack of energy, tiredness, weight loss of 2 stones, anorexia, cold hands, sweating and paraesthesia in the fingers – all of about 1 month duration. She was pale and dyspnoeic, the blood pressure was 100/60 mmHg and the pulse 120/minute.

Laboratory investigations

Initially, on 14.12.84, the serum sodium concentration was 129 mmol/l (RR 135–147), the serum potassium was 5.2 mmol/l (RR 3.5–5.0), the serum chloride 97 mmol/l (RR 95–107) and the serum bicarbonate 20.0 mmol/l (RR 21–30). The serum cortisol at 09.00 h on 17.12.84, prior to a tetracosactrin (Synacthen) stimulation test (short procedure), was 445 nmol/l (RR 221–773) with plasma ACTH values of 1974 and 2215 ng/l (RR < 10–80). The serum cortisol 30 min after the injection of 250 µg tetracosactrin intravenously was 396 nmol/l. The serum cortisol concentration on 19.12.84 was 291 nmol/l at 23.00 h, and 471 nmol/l prior to a repeat of the tetracosactrin stimulation test at 09.00 h on 20.12.84, the level 30 min later being 397 nmol/l. The serum free thyroxine (FT$_4$) value on 20.12.84 was 14.3 pmol/l (RR 9–28). Thyroid microsomal antibodies were reported positive to a titre of 1:6400 on 20.12.84, gastric parietal cell antibodies were positive to a titre of 1:1280 and adrenal cortex antibodies were also identified.

Date	Serum sodium (mmol/l)	Serum potassium (mmol/l)	Serum urea (mmol/l)	Serum creatinine (μmol/l)	Serum osmolality (mosmol/kg)	Urine sodium (mmol/l)
14.12.84	129	5.2	10.6	123	284	–
17.12.84	129	5.0	12.6	104	275	–
19.12.84	126	5.6	10.9	102	268	160
20.12.84	127	6.1	9.9	115	–	–
21.12.84	126	5.6	11.0	124	–	–
22.12.84	129	6.4	10.9	126	278	38
22.12.84	125	4.6	9.8	120	267	57
23.12.84	133	4.9	7.1	93	–	–
24.12.84	135	4.8	3.8	79	–	–
27.12.84	138	3.5	3.6	65	–	–
10.04.85	138	4.8	2.7	78	–	–
17.07.85	135	5.1	3.7	69	–	–
14.10.86	139	4.8	3.1	–	–	–

Analysis and comments

This patient was referred by the general practitioner to a physician on 14.12.84 with a one-month history of lack of energy, lassitude and anorexia; in recent weeks there had also been loss of 2 stones in weight. Apart from the lack of pigmentation these features are typical of Addison's disease. However, approximately 5% of such patients may lack pigmentation, which sometimes accounts for delay in establishing the diagnosis. Therapy with cortisone acetate in small dosage commenced late in the day on 20.12.84. Appetite and alertness improved dramatically within 3 h and her zest for life returned. On 22.12.84 the cortisone was increased to 30 mg b.d. and intravenous N saline was given to a total of 5.0 l over 48 h; oral fludrocortisone was also administered. On 24.12.84 the dose of cortisone was raised to 50 mg b.d. for a few days.

It was at her next out-patient appointment, a few weeks later, that she brought to attention for the first time her 2-year history of depression, for which neither she nor her mother had adequate explanation. Following the diagnosis of Addison's disease and the commencement of therapy, she said that the depression disappeared and she was absolutely certain that she would never again need any of her antidepressant medications; so confident was she that she had discarded her tablets 'down the loo'. She had not reported the depression earlier as it had not seemed relevant, only recognizing its full significance after it had dramatically disappeared following therapy. She said that she had 'forgotten what it was like to feel well'.

However, 12 months later she became unwell commencing with a mild upper respiratory tract infection and was instructed to double her cortisone dosage, but in view of the further development of wheeziness she was given oxytetracycline. One month later the depression returned and her cortisone dose was increased yet further for a short while, but with only slight improvement. The blood pressure was 110/70 mmHg. Although the cortisone was soon reduced the depression persisted. She admitted that she was thoroughly fed up with her present job and discussed whether she should change her occupation. At this point she was referred to a physician who performed thyroid function tests. Her serum free thyroxine (FT_4) was 10.0 pmol/l (RR 9–28) and her serum TSH 32.2 mU/l (RR < 5.5). These figures compare with a serum FT_4 of 14.3 pmol/l just 14 months earlier on 20.12.84, with a positive thyroid microsomal antibody titre of 1:6400. She was now clearly hypothyroid and was accordingly treated with thyroxine commencing with a dose of 50 μg/day, increasing at fortnightly intervals. She improved rapidly and the depression waned. On 18.06.87 the serum FT_4 was 23.8 pmol/l and the serum TSH < 0.08 mU/l; however, on 20.06.88 the serum FT_4 had risen to 29.6 pmol/l (RR 10.4–24.2) and the serum TSH was reduced to 0.18 mU/l (RR 0.44–3.16); a different range is quoted here because the laboratory method of analysis had changed. She was clinically hyperthyroid at this point, complaining of panic attacks on going out, particularly if far from home. Attention was paid to stabilizing her medication, therefore, because it became evident that there was a compliance problem. On 27.02.89 her serum FT_4 was 20.7 pmol/l and the TSH 4.1 mU/l. She has never had any recurrence of depression in the 8 years that have elapsed since that time; she continues to take steroid and thyroxine therapy – and confesses to feeling extremely well.

There is clearly a tendency to autoimmune disease in this patient. A paternal aunt had thyroid microsomal antibodies to a titre of 1:1600 and a maternal aunt likewise. Besides the Addison's disease and hypothyroidism, she is a potential subject for pernicious anaemia, premature ovarian failure, idiopathic hypoparathyroidism, vitiligo and insulin-dependent diabetes mellitus. It is imperative that she be observed carefully for the onset of pernicious anaemia, which could perhaps be accompanied, or even preceded, by depression in view of her past history. The arrangement is that she will be seen yearly should she not attend her general practitioner at an earlier date for any other reason.

Phaeochromocytoma[62,65]

Clinical aspects

The biological presentation of a phaeochromocytoma, whether it be located within the adrenal medulla, ectopically situated in relation to the sympathetic ganglia, part of the multiple endocrine neoplasia (MEN) syndrome (MEN type II, Sipple's syndrome) or as a component of von Recklinghausen's neurofibromatosis, comprises hypertension, profuse sweating, palpitations, pallor or flushing, and sometimes nausea and/or vomiting and diabetes mellitus; the symptoms may be either episodic or permanent. There is usually some mental accompaniment, however, taking the form of anxiety, intense fear, apprehension or a feeling of impending doom (angor animi). Attacks can last for a few minutes or even a few hours; as the disease advances, however, they increase in frequency, duration and severity. After an attack the patient may suffer excitability or confusion and then feel exhausted for several hours or days. Not all attacks are severe, and some consist only of feelings of faintness and mild anxiety. The close relatives and even the patient may regard such symptoms as being neurotic. Phaeochromocytomas are generally slow-growing tumours and some may have remained undiagnosed for in excess of 10 years. Should the tumour be sited in the urinary bladder it may present clinically with headache and the other symptoms already described, episodically – every time urine is voided.

Biochemical basis

These tumours synthesize, store and secrete catecholamines; the latter are not released, however, by way of neural stimulation as there is no innervation of these tumours. Both NA and adrenaline are secreted by most tumours. NA is the main secretion of the tumours of extra-adrenal origin, but occasionally adrenaline is the sole secretion (e.g. particularly in association with the MEN syndrome).

CASE 3[68]

Clinical history

A 65-year-old lady doctor, hitherto active, healthy and athletic, began in 1972 to develop palpitations and noticed mild attacks of arrhythmia, dyspnoea, headache and general feelings of being unwell. Her blood pressure was not raised and the ECG was normal. A viral infection was considered to be the likely diagnosis. The symptoms persisted over the next 3 years, at which time she developed a series of attacks of arrhythmia, each followed by a severe headache. The headaches became a regular feature and the attacks of arrhythmia were often precipitated by lying on the left side. She was frequently told that she looked grey and tired. She complained of vertigo, facial pain, dyspepsia and sudden attacks of diarrhoea. Her general practitioner referred her to an endocrinologist and a cardiologist, but both explained to her that there was no evidence of physical illness; she was found to be euthyroid. Her blood pressure readings were almost always normal, although they were slightly raised on two occasions. She then began to sweat more than normal and developed a slight tremor, which prevented her from playing the piano properly. Some of her colleagues considered her to be neurotic. By the end of the summer the headaches were worse; she complained of pulsation in the head, eyes and finger tips. Pentazocine was prescribed for the increasing pain. She was no longer able to lie down and the symptoms increased; she began to have to sleep in a chair until the early morning. Her life had changed completely. She became weak and ill during the day, was unable to undertake her normal activities and now found it impossible to do gardening because bending caused her head to ache; her consumption of pills and potions increased. The patient was again referred to the cardiologist who assured her that there was nothing wrong. In 1976 she began to feel

---

desperate, was almost suicidal and recognized that she was deteriorating; she was at a complete loss to explain her complaints. It then dawned on her that she might have a phaeochromocytoma. Cardiac monitoring during the night in hospital revealed multiple atrial ectopic beats. 'Wonderful relief' followed administration of a β-adrenoreceptor blocking drug.

Laboratory investigations

The 24 h urinary excretion of vanillylmandelic acid (VMA) was found to be elevated. Later, venous sampling *via* a femoral vein catheter revealed elevated catecholamine values in blood from the right renal vein. Retroperitoneal nitrogen insufflation demonstrated a tumour lying at the upper pole of the right kidney. At operation a tumour the size of a small orange was found in the right adrenal gland.

Analysis and comments

Following surgical removal of the phaeochromocytoma from the right adrenal gland the 24 h urinary VMA excretions fell markedly and now bordered on the upper end of the reference range. However, the postoperative course was not straightforward and there were many problems, although these are not relevant from the point of view of this discussion.

Phaeochromocytomas grow slowly and the symptoms develop insidiously. Apart from diabetes mellitus and hypertension (and its consequences) there can be attacks of anxiety, confusion, paranoia, depression and aggression; postoperatively there can be a dramatic change in mental attitude with loss of depression, aggression and paranoia. It is quite possible for a patient with severe psychiatric disturbance and a past history of suicide attempts to regress rapidly and completely following surgical removal of such a tumour.

Hypopituitarism[62]

Clinical aspects

There are many possible causes of hypopituitarism, some disorders involving just one pituitary hormone, whereas others involve two or more. Clinically, the presentation can either be acute or of insidious progression over many years. The majority of patients have at least some psychiatric component, with depression being particularly prominent. Often there is apathy, anergia, lethargy, drowsiness, and lack of initiative, with drift towards self-neglect, indifference, stupor and finally coma. In contrast to these features, irritability is sometimes seen, with episodes of delirium and, rarely, hallucinations. Memory impairment also occurs. Hypopituitarism, as is also the case with Addison's disease, is not often associated with a functional psychosis; on the other hand, acute organic reactions are not uncommonly seen in association with the metabolic disturbance. There is the danger of coma on rare occasions when there are stressful biological events (e.g. infection, hypoglycaemia, etc.).

Biochemical basis

Deficiencies of ACTH (with its consequential reduction of adrenocortical activity), TSH (leading to hypothyroidism) and FSH and LH (leading to sex hormone depletion) are the main hormonal abnormalities upon which other biochemical disturbances are founded; the psychiatric features are secondary to these.

METABOLIC ENCEPHALOPATHIES

In this section, opportunity will be taken to discuss blood gas disturbances and hypoglycaemia, together with disorders of the liver and kidney, all of which have wide-ranging cerebral metabolic implications. The metabolic consequences of alcohol intoxication, too, will be included here.

Hypoxia[4,69-71]

Clinical aspects

Inattentiveness and defects of judgement characterize mild hypoxia; more severe depletion can cause coma in as little time as 10 sec, although if O_2 is given within 4 min the process is completely reversible. Should the O_2 lack be for a longer period then irreparable damage ensues, affecting particularly the globus pallidus, hippocampus and parts of the parieto-occipital cortex. Persistent severe hypoxia leads to a decerebrate state, but should the patient recover then confusion or dementia may remain.

Anoxic/ischaemic encephalopathy can be caused by local pathology (e.g. cerebral thrombosis, embolus or haemorrhage), or by lesions outside the CNS – such as those of cardiac origin (e.g. myocardial infarction, cardiac arrest, congestive cardiac failure, etc.), shock (e.g. haemorrhagic, infective, traumatic) and respiratory problems, e.g. suffocation, paralysis of respiratory muscles and carbon monoxide (CO) poisoning, etc.

Biochemical basis

The O_2 content of room air is normally 20.93%, but if the value falls there is then compensatory increased cerebral blood flow in order to maintain tissue supply. The O_2 content of air can fall, however, to 10% before any noticeable behavioural effects are seen; should it drop to 7% then there is increased glycolysis and a 300% increase in lactate formation – although energy production in the form of ATP is maintained. Mild hypoxia decreases the activity of aromatic amine hydroxylases, thereby causing interference with DA, NA and 5HT synthesis. Continued hypoxia leads to impaired energy production, secondarily affecting electrolyte transport and repolarization; finally, there is structural damage to the mitochondria.

CASE 4[72]

Clinical history

A 40-year-old man was reported by his wife to have been unconscious for 3 h and to be breathing intermittently. The lady had rung the general practitioner at 01.30 h saying slowly 'My husband has been unconscious for 3 h and stops breathing now and then – do you think he is alright?'. It was a cold, dark and stormy night as the doctor arrived at the house, knocked at the door and, finding it to be unlatched, entered a very untidy kitchen. A young lady, looking pale and ill, slowly stood up and explained that she had been 'very sick'; there was vomit all over her jumper, her hair and the floor. Her husband, however, was clearly the main concern, because he was lying face downwards on the floor between the kitchen and dining room, deeply unconscious and with contracted pupils; there was no evidence of violence, alcohol or drugs. His ruddy complexion befitted an outdoor occupation. The respiration rate was slow, but his

---

pulse was normal. His wife said that he had not taken any medications and that he was normally in excellent health; indeed, only the week before he had passed his annual medical examination, confirming that he was fit to continue flying as a pilot.

Admission to hospital was arranged immediately, but whilst awaiting the ambulance the doctor listened further to the wife's story; she observed that she spoke very slowly, sounding rather like a 'zombie'. It appeared that at 21.00 h she recalled that her husband was quite well. However, she remembered nothing else up to 01.30 h when she telephoned the doctor seeking help. Accordingly, the lady too, was advised to go to hospital with her husband for a check-up. Whilst she was preparing herself, the doctor observed the cats to be scampering around; 'no signs of lethargy there!', she thought.

Laboratory investigations

Twenty-four hours later the carboxyhaemoglobin level was found to be markedly raised in the man's blood; a lesser level, although also raised, was found in the case of the lady.

Analysis and comments

The man was fully conscious 12 h later following the administration of oxygen. At interview one week afterwards he was able to give the following story. He had found his wife in a fainting state, and accordingly had managed to drag her towards the ill-fitting door of the kitchen, under which a draught happened to be blowing. This presumably enabled her to survive and revive by keeping the high concentration of CO away from her. With the considerable effort involved he had lost consciousness himself, ending up lying face down. With the high concentration of gas around him he had thus become asphyxiated. The extraordinary thing was that the wife, in her stuporous state, was able to telephone the doctor. On investigation, the source of CO was found to be the Rayburn heater, which was faulty; it was, therefore, immediately removed. The outcome was fortunate in that neither husband nor wife suffered permanent brain damage; he was soon back working as an aircraft pilot. The cats seemed to have escaped obvious damage by jumping on the table and chairs.

Inhalation of a low concentration of CO (e.g. 0.01% CO in air) will produce a carboxyhaemoglobin concentration of < 10%, normally without any clinical symptoms, whereas inhalation of 0.05% for 1 h, together with just light activity, will lead to a blood carboxyhaemoglobin concentration of 20%. There is, associated with this, a mild throbbing headache and perhaps exertional dyspnoea. Greater activity or longer exposure to the same concentration will produce a blood carboxyhaemoglobin of 30–50%, with headache, irritability, confusion, dizziness, visual disturbance, nausea, vomiting and fainting on exertion. Exposure to 0.1% CO in air leads to a carboxyhaemoglobin concentration in the blood of 50–80%. There would then be coma, convulsions and cardiorespiratory arrest – and finally, death. However, should a very high concentration of CO be inhaled, then there could be very rapid saturation of the blood together with rapid loss of consciousness without the usual preceding symptoms. There is a cherry red colour when the skin and mucosae are examined, but this is not always easy to detect. The development of neuropsychiatric problems may occur a number of weeks after recovery from CO poisoning. There can be impairment of memory, deterioration of intellect, and personality change (irritability, verbal aggressiveness, violence, impulsiveness and mood variability).

Hypercapnia[71]

Clinical aspects

If CO_2 retention is of acute onset, or if there is an acute exacerbation of chronic hypercapnia, then intense and persistent headache develops, accompanied by inattention and indifference to events in the environment. There is also weakness, irritability and lassitude, progressing to drowsiness, confusion, stupor and coma. Causes include various chronic pulmonary disorders, e.g. chronic emphysema and chronic fibrosing lung disease. Entry to a high CO_2 containing atmosphere would produce rapid coma and death.

Biochemical basis

CO_2 narcosis (as part of chronic respiratory acidosis) is the basis of the situation, together with secondary polycythaemia and cerebral vasodilatation. If there is inadequate central respiratory drive, the arterial blood PCO_2 rises and the PO_2 falls. If hypoxaemia and hypercapnia occur simultaneously the neurological effects of each may be indistinguishable. Chronic hypercapnia will produce no symptomatology if the respiratory acidosis is fully compensated. Lung infection, if present, would further worsen the biochemical and clinical presentation.

Hyperventilation syndrome[73]

Clinical aspects

The patient with this disorder is most likely to be an anxious female who, although being unaware of overbreathing, might admit to sighing and feeling apprehensive. Nevertheless, anxiety does not seem to be prerequisite for the disorder, as chronic hyperventilation is reported to occur in the absence of overt anxiety. In the acute disorder light-headedness is typical and panic attacks occur either for no very obvious reason, or in some instances, may be provoked by identifiable circumstances. In the chronic disorder there are feelings of unreality, difficulties in concentrating, anxiety and attacks of panic; an interesting feature is that symptoms are sometimes more marked at rest than during moderate exercise. Apart from the hyperventilation syndrome, a number of other disorders can cause hypocapnia – including mild asthma, chronic pulmonary disease, congestive cardiac failure, pulmonary emboli and severe pain.

Biochemical basis

In acute hyperventilation the arterial PCO_2 is reduced without any change in the plasma bicarbonate as there has been insufficient time for compensatory processes to take place. In chronic hyperventilation there is compensated respiratory alkalosis; both the arterial PCO_2 and the plasma bicarbonate are reduced, but there is a relatively normal blood pH. The low arterial PCO_2 may account for neuronal hyperexcitability and vasoconstriction, with consequent reduction in cerebral blood flow, possibly accounting for the fainting, giddiness and blurred vision so often observed. Adrenaline release may be the basis for some of the cardiovascular symptomatology in these patients.

Hypoglycaemia[5,70,71]

Clinical aspects

Prior to discussing neuropsychiatric implications, hypoglycaemia should first be defined as an arterial plasma glucose level of <2.2 mmol/l, although this would not necessarily be accompanied by cerebral symptoms (i.e. neuroglycopenia). In addition, should there have been a very rapid fall of glucose concentration from a high value then neuroglycopenia could occur even at a value of >2.2 mmol/l. A steady state value for plasma glucose of 2.2 mmol/l would, moreover, not necessarily equate with neuroglycopenia, as tissues can accommodate to such a situation. Of note is the fact that the infant brain is less susceptible to hypoglycaemia than the adult brain. It is, therefore, not only the blood glucose level itself that must be taken into account in any clinical situation, but also the rate of change.

The mood changes of neuroglycopenia comprise lethargy, lack of concentration, poor judgement, faintness and dizziness; the condition may proceed further to convulsions and coma. If, however, the blood glucose has fallen very rapidly the sympathetic nervous system may be stimulated, with the result that there is agitation, tremor, sweating, tachycardia, palpitations and pallor.

Hypoglycaemia can be classified as fasting or reactive. Fasting hypoglycaemia occurs where there is imbalance between hepatic glucose production and peripheral tissue utilization. In some cases there is defective glucose production (e.g. hypopituitarism, Addison's disease, glycogen synthetase deficiency, ketotic hypoglycaemia of infancy, severe malnutrition, acquired liver disease, alcohol ingestion, etc.), whereas in others there is excessive glucose utilization (e.g. insulinoma, insulin administration, sulphonylurea dosage, etc.). Reactive hypoglycaemia occurs postprandially; causes include partial gastrectomy, hereditary fructose intolerance, galactosaemia, leucine sensitivity, etc.

Biochemical basis

The tissues of the brain possess a very high metabolic rate, both during wakefulness and in sleep. This constant requirement for energy by the brain is approximately 1700 kJ (405 kcal) per day, representing about 20–25% of the total energy needs of a normal resting adult. This high need for energy is supplied almost entirely by the metabolic conversion of approximately 120 g glucose each day to CO_2, H_2O and energy. The ketones, 3-hydroxybutyrate and acetoacetate, can also be utilized in small amounts, but glycogen is not available in sufficient quantities to be an important source of energy. The brain is neither able to store nor synthesize glucose; moreover, the entry of glucose to the brain is not under hormonal control. There is, therefore, heavy reliance on the glucose content of the extracellular fluid. Hence, significant hypoglycaemia is able to markedly impair neuronal function. If hypoglycaemic encephalopathy persists for many minutes there is exhaustion of the cerebral glucose reserve; cerebral oxidation then proceeds in the absence of exogenous glucose, with the result that neuronal lipid and protein is metabolized; hence, irreversible damage occurs.

CASE 5

Clinical history

A 68-year-old lady had attended a medical clinic regularly on account of hypertension since 1971. Her original blood pressure recording was 240/130 mmHg, but following therapy it had varied around 170/100 mmHg. Nine years later, on 25.04.80, a consultant neurologist was asked to see her; he noted that her current therapy comprised bendrofluazide 10 mg/day, although she had had guanethidine and propanolol in the past. He also noted that these treatments had been limited on account of numerous attacks of dizziness, nausea and vertigo associated with sweating and feeling hot. She had even had to be admitted to hospital for such episodes, although no satisfactory explanation had been forthcoming. The view taken was that a major part of her problem was anxiety, because in this context it was known that a good deal of panic was provoked at home whenever she complained of dizziness. Accordingly, he felt there was likely to be a real risk of unnecessary chronic invalidism – and of valium dependency, too, should that be prescribed. No further out-patient appointment was made.

On 07.05.80 her general practitioner wrote that the patient complained of attacks of shaking which prevented her from going out and also curtailed her otherwise, up to now, acceptably normal life. She said that these episodes were preceded by 'a grey blob in my mind, outlined by a golden colour', and that she had to hold her head until this

---

feeling went, usually lasting about 15 min. A nurse who happened to witness an attack one day when the patient was in the general practitioner's surgery said that she went bright red and hot and all four limbs started shaking, although she remained fully conscious. Accordingly, another neurological opinion was sought.

On 10.07.80 the second consultant neurologist extracted a detailed history, commenting that this seemed to be a formidable problem for diagnosis. It appeared that she had had repeated shaking attacks over the last 4–5 years, occurring invariably if she went outside, and up to 2–3 times/week. The attacks often came in the morning with the grey blob in her field of vision, which developed a golden edge, lasting for 15–20 min. She became exhausted after this, her head felt as if it was on fire, she perspired and then started shaking 'from top to bottom'. The shaking commenced at the top of her head, going through to her feet and lasting 15–30 min. Her husband, who witnessed some of these attacks, confirmed that she had to hang on to the bed-rail sometimes whilst she was shaking; there was no loss of consciousness, however, on these occasions, though perhaps she was a 'little bit out of contact'. In addition, the husband said that she had had one attack of loss of consciousness lasting at least 30 min and because of this was taken to the local hospital. Her blood pressure was found to be 210/130 mmHg and she was advised to re-commence the bendrofluazide which had, it seems, been stopped. It was again considered likely that these attacks were epileptic in nature, but there was also recognized to be considerable anxiety on account of her having become house-bound. An electroencephalogram (EEG), performed on 14.08.80, was reported as showing 'a generalized abnormality of non-specific nature, which would certainly be compatible with an epileptic basis for her attacks, though it is not diagnostic of epilepsy'. Various drugs were suggested, including carbamazepine and propanolol. No further appointment was made.

Sixteen months later, on 04.11.81, following an episode of coma, the general practitioner referred her to a consultant physician for assessment of the same general problem. He added the observation that the carbamazepine she had previously been given had altered the lady's blackouts in that she was now having less shaking and that the pre-ictal symptoms of spots before the eyes had improved. Her husband provided the information that the fits would very likely occur when she was going to face a stressful situation – such as visiting the out-patients department to see the consultant. She was at this point admitted to hospital for further observation and investigations.

This provided the opportunity for a yet more detailed history of her complaints, which were now of 10 years duration, to be taken. Commencing in about 1972, there had been a progressive onset of grey blobs in her visual field, each with a golden edge, fading later to green. These attacks came frequently. In the first 2 years of her illness she sometimes felt ravenously hungry after the blobs had appeared; in the last 8 years hunger no longer occurred. On one occasion she bought a quarter of a pound of cheese from a shop and ate it all whilst walking along the street in order to alleviate her unpleasant feelings. After the blobs had disappeared she sometimes used to see '2–3 of everything' around her, e.g. wardrobes, plants – and even husbands! Moreover, she was unable to focus her eyes properly on television for up to several hours. She said she used to get a tremor in her body from head to toe; she realized this would not be noticeable to others, but she was intensely aware of it herself. After these episodes she became exhausted and sweated profusely – but only at the back of the head which became soaking wet; the sweating involved no other part of the body. She commented that the doctors had said that there was nothing they could do to help her. The blackouts first started in 1973, but became more frequent in recent years lasting from 20 min for up to 3 h; they came every day latterly and were unrelated to food. She could be quietly sitting at a table and then would be unconscious a few minutes later; she would wake up with the neighbours on each side of her. Her husband said it was all very frightening. She said 'will I ever get right again?'. Furthermore, she had had unsteadiness of gait since a recent fall, and sometimes she felt as if the room was going round her. The attacks of loss of consciousness were followed by a feeling of tightness in the head.

Laboratory investigations

Date	Time (24 h)	Blood glucose (mmol/l)	Serum insulin (mU/l)	Serum C-peptide (µg/l)	Clinical observations
01.12.81	13.45	5.0	26.6	1.6	
01.12.81	14.45	2.8	15.0	–	
07.12.81	–	1.5	32.3	1.7	72 h fast commences
07.12.81	11.45	1.8	36.6	1.5	
07.12.81	15.30	3.0	12.7	1.2	
07.12.81	23.15	1.5	–	–	Sudden faintness, face feels flushed

Continued

Laboratory investigations continued

Date	Time (24 h)	Blood glucose (mmol/l)	Serum insulin (mU/l)	Serum C-peptide (µg/l)	Clinical observations
					grey blobs visually, sweating profusely. 50 ml 50% dextrose iv
08.12.81	00.30	2.0	–	–	5% dextrose iv
08.12.81	06.00	4.0	–	–	Headache
08.12.81	09.00	–	–	–	Drip to come down, fasting to continue
08.12.81	09.30	2.8	30.5	–	
08.12.81	17.00	3.3	12.5	–	
09.12.81	16.00	1.5	–	–	Talking 'rubbish', cold, sweating, blurred vision,
09.12.81	16.20	2.0	11.9	1.2	
09.12.81	23.00	1.5	–	–	Blurred vision, cold, sweating, slurred speech
10.12.81	04.00	1.5	–	–	Drowsiness increasing, slurred speech, responding to questions, no longer sweating
10.12.81	07.15	2.0	8.8	1.1	Suddenly unresponsive to commands and no response to painful stimuli, eyes glazed, no actual fit observed. 50 ml 50% dextrose iv
10.12.81	07.45	–	–	–	Much improved and talking sensibly
10.12.81	–	1.3	15.6	1.5	Permitted to eat again.
14.12.81	–	7.8	–	–	Therapy with diazoxide and chlorothiazide

Analysis and comments

This patient, with a history of a complex and progressive illness, had a story which unfolded further at each consultation. Although the story was available for the asking, it was viewed in a different context on each occasion, with the emphasis of questioning being directed one way or the other according to the interests and expertise of the physician and the time available for establishing the correct sequence of events. It is always easy in retrospect to see the whole, but the actual route by which the diagnosis was eventually made was via the general practitioner who arranged a blood glucose analysis at the time of seeing her in coma, the value for which was 2.0 mmol/l; this aroused suspicion of hypoglycaemia due to an insulinoma. Soon after this, on 04.11.81, the letter of referral to the consultant physician was sent.

This was not the first time an insulinoma had been considered; it was, in fact, thought of at the first neurological consultation, but the correct procedure of investigation had not been pursued. If a fasting test of 72 h duration had been arranged, together with serial blood glucose and serum insulin and C-peptide values, then the diagnosis should have been made at that time. However, it was some 20 months later that this test was done and which finally confirmed the nature of the condition. There was inappropriate presence of serum insulin and C-peptide at the time of symptomatic hypoglycaemia. Nevertheless, the hazards of removing an insulinoma in a lady of this age should not be overlooked. There is no merit in making such a diagnosis only to find that some serious complication has arisen or death has occurred. She was accordingly treated with diazoxide and chlorothiazide. Within 24 h she had made a dramatic recovery and was able to fully reflect on her story and present it articulately.

This lady possessed a small physical lesion in the pancreas (an insulinoma) which produced a chemical secretion (insulin), with biological consequences (hypoglycaemia), producing psychological sequelae, and sociological implications, too. There was destruction of the family life – the neighbours no longer wished to come and see her, nor did the lady wish to be seen by them, and her husband gave up his job in order to look after her. All this 'melted away' within 24 h following institution of the correct therapy. She enthusiastically said 'life has begun all over again after 10 years of misery'. She has remained completely well whilst continuing therapy during the succeeding 15 years.

Hyperglycaemia[70,71]

Clinical aspects

The acute metabolic complications of diabetes mellitus are diabetic ketoacidosis and hyperosmolar coma. In both situations there is hyperglycaemia; however, in the former condition, associated with type 1 diabetes mellitus (insulin-dependent diabetes mellitus, IDDM), keto-acidosis is dominant – with the hyperglycaemia sometimes being of minimal degree, whereas in the latter, associated with type 2 diabetes mellitus (non-insulin-dependent diabetes mellitus, NIDDM), there is no metabolic acidosis – but the hyperglycaemia is gross.

In diabetic ketoacidosis there is anorexia, nausea, vomiting, polyuria, polydipsia and abdominal pain; if the condition remained untreated then impairment of consciousness would result, with progression to coma.

Hyperosmolar non-ketotic diabetic coma is secondary to the severe dehydration that would occur on account of polyuria (secondary to rising hyperglycaemia), should there also be failure to drink sufficient water to maintain fluid balance. The disorder usually occurs in elderly people, either living alone or who may not be receiving adequate medical/nursing care. Common precipitating factors include cerebral thrombosis, infection, etc. A clouding of consciousness, progressing later to coma, comprises the neuropsychiatric presentation. It is the lack of development of the unpleasant symptoms of ketoacidosis that opens the way for there being serious delay in bringing the patient to medical attention, thus permitting dehydration to achieve a more severe degree.

Biochemical basis

It is essentially the elevated plasma levels of acetoacetate and β-hydroxybutyrate, together with a lesser contribution from the rise of lactate, fatty acids and phosphates, that accounts for the metabolic acidosis of IDDM. Prior to the clinical presentation of the ketoacidosis there will have been polyuria, with loss of electrolytes (particularly potassium and phosphate) – hence, depletion of body potassium and phosphate, even though serum levels of these substances may, at presentation, be either within their reference ranges or actually elevated. In addition, magnesium deficiency may be present. Serum sodium concentrations tend to be low, secondary to the dilutional osmotic effects of glucose which draws fluid from the intracellular compartment to the plasma.

In the hyperosmolar state the extreme hyperglycaemia, elevated plasma viscosity, plasma hyperosmolality, volume depletion, dehydration and consequent pre-renal uraemia all have their impact on cerebral function. In those patients who do not survive, evidence of disseminated intravascular coagulation may be found in the brain at postmortem examination.

Hepatic failure[69-71]

Clinical aspects

Hepatic encephalopathy is characterized, apart from other clinical symptoms and signs, by episodes ranging from mild mental dulling to increased or decreased psychomotor activity, confusion, drowsiness and coma.

Acute hepatic encephalopathy can unfold over a few days or weeks. It may be caused by acute infectious hepatitis, drug toxicity (e.g. paracetamol overdose), ingestion of poisons (e.g. carbon tetrachloride), the various hyperammonaemic syndromes seen in childhood and Reye's syndrome (which is accompanied by hepatic enlargement and marked cerebral oedema). Chronic hepatic insufficiency with portacaval shunting of blood, chronic alcoholic cirrhosis and chronic hepatitis of other causes can all be the basis of hepatic encephalopathy. Neuropathologically, hepatic coma is characterized by an increase in both the number and size of the protoplasmic astrocytes in the cerebral cortex.

Biochemical basis

There is still conjecture as to the biochemical basis of the condition. Nevertheless, it is established that cerebral oxidative metabolism is impaired, with both O_2 uptake and glucose utilization being reduced – although such changes might be consequential rather than causal.

Ammonia (NH_3), formed from the breakdown of amino acids or (together with other amines) derived from gastrointestinal urease-containing organisms, is normally converted to urea. In hepatic failure or in the presence of a portacaval shunt, however, the NH_3 and amines cannot be converted to urea and hence continue to circulate to all organs including the brain. The synergism of action of certain metabolites (e.g. fatty acids, methyl mercaptan and NH_3) could, in part, be the basis of hepatic encephalopathy.

Hepatic encephalopathy could also be accounted for by changes in the synthesis and metabolism of neurotransmitters, or perhaps because of the presence of false neurotransmitters (e.g. octopamine and phenylethanolamine). It is well established that plasma amino acids are abnormal in hepatic disease; aromatic amino acids in particular enter the brain in greater amounts than normal, possibly leading to changes in neurotransmitter synthesis (e.g. increase in 5HT and β-hydroxyphenylethanolamines). A rise in the amount of the inhibitory neurotransmitter, GABA, has also been suggested as being an explanation for the mental sequelae of hepatic disease.

Uraemia[69,71]

Clinical aspects

Initially, the psychiatric manifestations of acute uraemic encephalopathy comprise apathy, fatigue, inattentiveness and irritability. Later, there is confusion, hallucinations, stupor and coma. These features are sometimes episodic. In the 'disequilibrium syndrome', which sometimes complicates haemodialysis or peritoneal dialysis, the patient develops headaches, irritability, agitation, drowsiness and convulsions, commencing several hours following the onset of dialysis (occasionally up to 2 days after the procedure) and of several hours duration. There is also a less common manifestation, 'dialysis encephalopathy', in which there is a change of personality and episodes of psychosis with intellectual decline. At first these episodes last for a few hours and occur soon after dialysis but later, as they progress, they become more persistent and finally achieve permanency.

There are many causes of renal failure, but special mention should be made of the difficulties sometimes encountered in separating the renal failure itself from the disease which caused it (e.g. hypertension can itself cause hypertensive encephalopathy, whereas the consequent renal failure can also produce an encephalopathy of its own).

Neuropathologically, there is in some cases hyperplasia of the protoplasmic astrocytes in the cerebral cortex, but to a much lesser degree than that seen in hepatic encephalopathy. Cerebral oedema is characteristically absent.

Biochemical basis

There are a multitude of biochemical changes in renal failure; nevertheless, the rise of blood urea and creatinine are not the basis of the mental features. There is, however, a 30% reduction in O_2 utilization by the brain, but without any change in cerebral circulation. Glucose consumption by the brain is decreased; this, together with the elevated ATP and phosphocreatine levels in the brain, implies some defect in energy utilization. The anaerobic metabolism of pyruvate causes an increase of acetoin and 2,3-butyleneglycol.

In chronic renal failure, the electrolyte imbalance, acid–base disturbance and toxin accumulation leads to defective ion transportation across cell membranes. The latter, in turn, leads to alteration in the ionic composition of intracellular and extracellular fluids. The normal active transportation of Na^+ out of the cells to the surrounding fluid medium is metabolically costly, accounting for a significantly large proportion of basal energy utilization and O_2 consumption. In the brain tissue of uraemic patients there is found to be a reduction in Na^+ and K^+ stimulated ATPase activity. It is probable, ultimately, that a defect in membrane polarization accounts for the neuropsychiatric changes.

In the disequilibrium syndrome there is a shift of water into the brain tissues. Dialysis encephalopathy is characterized by mild diffuse microcavitation of the upper layers of the cerebral cortex. Aluminium has been found in higher amounts in the cerebral grey matter of such patients when compared with those who were dialysed but who did not have encephalopathy. The aluminium is derived not only from dialysate fluid but also from orally administered aluminium containing gels. It has been suggested, therefore, that aluminium intoxication might possibly be the basis of these disorders.

Ethyl alcohol[74–80]

Clinical aspects

Alcohol ingestion produces mood changes and neuropsychiatric symptoms which vary according to circumstances. Alcohol toxicity in the short-term is associated, initially, with progression from inebriation to the slowing of thought processes, being unable to concentrate, and displaying an unreliable memory, loss of restraint, irregular behaviour, drowsiness – and finally coma. Should 'pathological intoxication' occur then irrational outbursts of anger (with the accompanying danger of physical violence) may be expressed. 'Alcoholic blackouts' may take the form of amnesia for significant events taking place during the bout of drinking, lasting from a few hours up to several days; subsequent exposure to alcohol may aid recall of those events. Hypoglycaemia, symptomatic or asymptomatic, sometimes occurs – commencing a few hours after the alcohol ingestion, lasting even for 36 h or more. There may be long-term complications such as the neuropsychiatric accompaniments of cirrhosis of the liver or severe hepatitis. The nutritional consequences of alcohol ingestion comprise vitamin B_1 deficiency and the consequent Wernicke's encephalopathy and Korsakoff's psychosis. Alcohol may also induce falls and head injuries; it is always important to consider taking an x-ray of the skull or doing a computerized tomography (CT) scan. The administration of certain drugs concomitantly with the alcohol (e.g. benzodiazepines, barbiturates, etc.) can produce dangerously high drug levels in the blood, with profound clinical consequences. Withdrawal of alcohol leads to fits, hallucinations and delirium tremens. Chronic alcoholics occasionally develop Cushing's syndrome, although withdrawal of alcohol usually leads to quick resolution of the features in a few days or weeks. All these factors, individually or combined, are yet further influenced by the personality of the individual, the mood of the moment, the company that is being kept, the culture of origin and genetic inheritance.

Neuropathological changes occurring in patients with a high alcohol intake include slight reduction in the weight of the brain with increased pericerebral space, the changes of Wernicke's encephalopathy, cerebral atrophy of the dorso-lateral aspect of the frontal lobes in particular, and enlargement of the frontal horns of the lateral ventricles. Histologically, there is arachnoidal thickening and cell degeneration with partial destruction of the myelin sheath.

Approximately 70% or more of ingested alcohol, assuming that the serum alcohol concentration does not exceed 20 mmol/l (92 mg/100 ml), is metabolized in the liver *via* alcohol dehydrogenase to acetaldehyde, which is then converted by aldehyde dehydrogenase to acetate. Both enzymes require NAD as cofactor, NADH being produced in the process. Hence, the ratio NADH:NAD rises – which, in turn, influences the rate of activity of other metabolic reactions. This ratio is responsible, therefore, for many of the metabolic derangements caused by high alcohol consumption. Should the alcohol in the blood rise higher, then the microsomal ethanol oxidizing system (MEOS) takes on a role of increasing importance, accounting for up to 10% or more of the metabolism of alcohol; this pathway is NADP dependent. There is a third pathway, too, which is involved in alcohol metabolism when levels are high, i.e. the catalase pathway.

In general, alcohol metabolism proceeds at around 10 ml/h in an adult if the serum alcohol level does not exceed 20 mmol/l; the reaction is, nevertheless, proportional to body weight and is also influenced by diurnal variation (i.e. the rate of metabolism is higher in the morning).

Oxidation of alcohol yields energy of 7.1 kcal/g (29.7 kJ/g), compared with approximate values for protein of 5.5 kcal/g (23.0 kJ/g), fat of 9.3 kcal/g (39.0 kJ/g) and carbohydrate of 4.0 kcal/g (16.8 kJ/g). As a result of high alcohol intake there is often concomitant reduction of nutritional intake, with development of negative nitrogen balance. Nevertheless, a high alcohol intake of 1000 kcal/day (4189 kJ/day) makes a significant contribution to the frequently seen weight gain in such patients.

Following oft repeated exposure to alcohol, however, various compensatory processes take place. Metabolic (pharmacokinetic) tolerance refers to increase in the rate of metabolism of alcohol, cellular (pharmacodynamic) tolerance concerns cell membrane and neurochemical adaptation, and behaviour tolerance involves the individual's ability to adapt and function better when there are higher levels of alcohol in the blood than would otherwise be expected.

A guide to the symptomatology to be expected with different serum alcohol levels is as follows: 20–30 mg/dl (4.4–6.5 mmol/l) – behavioural and cognitive changes commence at this level which may follow 1–2 drinks; 50–100 mg/dl (10.9–21.7 mmol/l) – flushing, slowing of the reflexes and impaired visual activity; 80 mg/l (17.4 mmol/l) – the legal limit for driving in the UK; 80–100 mg/dl (17.4–21.7 mmol/l) – 'intoxicated'; >100 mg/dl (>21.7 mmol/l) – depression of the CNS; 160 mg/dl (34.8 mmol/l) – narcosis, deep sleep; 300–400 mg/dl (65.2–87.0 mmol/l) – death, with or without other drugs complicating the issue.

Biochemical basis

Important observations relating alcohol metabolism to neuropsychiatric symptoms include the high NADH formation with consequential rise in the NADH:NAD ratio, the resulting inhibition of Kreb's cycle due to less NAD being available and inhibition of gluconeogenesis with transient hypoglycaemia of up to 36 h duration as outcome (exacerbated by accompanying poor nutritional intake and the possible presence of liver disease). Alcoholic ketoacidosis may occur and vitamin B_1 deficiency sometimes leads to Wernicke's encephalopathy and Korsakoff's psychosis, an increased lactate:pyruvate ratio and development of hyperlactataemia (with the danger of acid–base imbalance). Hypomagnesaemia may be a contributory factor to the clouding of consciousness, hypocalcaemia may contribute to weakness, and deficiency of zinc ions might be of importance in gonadal function.

Alcohol acts initially on the reticular formation in the brainstem, thereby stimulating increased excitability of the cerebral cortex. Following on from this, however, comes the direct toxic inhibitory action of the compound on the cerebral cortex. Alcohol is, therefore, a CNS depressant which causes inhibition of neuronal activity. Even moderate exposure to alcohol influences neurotransmitter systems. In 'alcoholic dementia' and cerebral atrophy, postmortem studies yield evidence for a reduction in cholinergic function, somewhat similar to the findings in Alzheimer's disease. Moreover, acetaldehyde formed during the metabolism of alcohol possesses toxic effects of its own; it is more toxic than alcohol and its effects are narcotic.

ELECTROLYTE AND WATER DISORDERS[69,71,81]

It must be emphasized that, in disorders of electrolyte and H_2O balance, it is by way of the accompanying osmolality disturbances that changes in brain volume determine, in general, the mode of clinical expression. Moreover, it is the sodium content of the different fluid compartments of the body that is the main contributor to their osmolality.

Water intoxication

Clinical aspects

This hypo-osmolar syndrome can be due to a number of factors, e.g. infusion post-operatively with low sodium-containing fluids, administration of analogues of antidiuretic hormone (ADH, vasopressin), compulsive H_2O drinking and the syndrome of inappropriate ADH (SIADH) secretion. In the early stages of H_2O intoxication the patient passes through a period of being less alert than usual, followed by lassitude, lethargy, apathy, restlessness, confusion, delirium, headache, stupor, convulsions and, eventually, coma. A slow fall in serum sodium concentration and osmolality permits accommodation to take place, whereas a rapid fall of values would lead to occurrence of symptoms at a higher level (at which none would normally be present). Compulsive H_2O drinking may be episodic. There is not only the consequential mood change, but also the psychiatric origin of the disorder to consider; thus the individual may be neurotic (e.g. anxiety state, etc.), psychotic (e.g. delusions, schizophrenia, etc.) or have a personality disorder (e.g. depression, hypochondria, etc.). There may be variation in fluid intake over the course of the day, unlike diabetes insipidus.

Biochemical basis

The extracellular fluid (ECF) osmolality falls, and the cell H_2O content rises on account of osmotic transference of fluid. The H_2O content of the brain as a whole, therefore, becomes markedly increased and the intracranial pressure rises. Therefore, the brain sodium and potassium concentrations fall, as the intracellular osmolality drops; the outcome could be cell membrane depolarization. There are contributions to the neurological features from both cell swelling and potassium changes.

CASE 6

Clinical history

A 29-year-old man had been a patient in a psychiatric hospital for about 2 years with a history of paranoid schizophrenia and multiple suicide attempts. He fell downstairs at 22.00 h on 23.06.88, sustaining a right-sided peri-orbital haematoma, shortly after which he was found cold, sweating and clammy, but fully conscious. Without delay he was referred to the accident and emergency department of the local general hospital where he was noted to be only partially alert. Whilst awaiting X-ray studies he had two grand mal epileptic fits, following which he became totally unconscious with a large dilated pupil on the left side; the right pupil could not be seen because of the peri-orbital haematoma. He was referred directly to the local neurosurgical unit in a comatose state, although no localizing signs were found; his CT scan, however, proved to be normal. He became restless and had to be nursed on a mattress on the floor for his own safety. Later, he improved and was able to respond to hearing his own name and to commands. He began to move both sides of his body and became more settled, more alert and less uncooperative.

Laboratory investigations

Date	Serum sodium (mmol/l)	Serum potassium (mmol/l)	Serum urea (mmol/l)	Serum osmolality (mosmol/kg)
13.04.73	135	–	4.5	–
02.08.83	141	4.2	4.8	–
05.11.84	137	4.0	2.4	–
24.06.88	104	3.3	1.5	–
24.06.88	109	3.5	–	–
24.06.88	112	3.3	1.6	–
24.06.88	123	4.3	2.8	250
25.06.88	125	4.7	5.3	253
26.06.88	126	3.7	7.9	259
27.06.88	130	4.5	6.3	–

Initially, on 24.06.88, the serum sodium concentration was 104 mmol/l (RR 135–147), the serum potassium level was 3.5 mmol/l (RR 3.5–5.0), the blood glucose 5.6 mmol/l (RR 3.0–6.0), the serum urea 2.8 mmol/l

(RR 2.0–6.5) and the serum creatinine 85 μmol/l (RR 44–123). The serum osmolality was recorded to be low at 250 mosmol/kg (RR 280–290) at a time when the serum sodium was 123 mmol/l. The serum calcium level, together with the urinary electrolytes and osmolality, are not available. There is no record of the patient's weight, and the fluid intake/urinary output chart was only recorded over a period of 3 days.

Analysis and comments

Soon after admission to the neurosurgical unit it was established that the serum sodium concentration was very low at 104 mmol/l (RR 135–147); it then emerged that he had a past history of psychogenic polydipsia. In the first 24 h he passed 8.0 l urine, during which time his serum sodium had risen from 104 to 112 mmol/l; concomitant with this rise was the improvement in conscious level already noted. His recent medications included chlorpromazine, procyclidine, phenytoin, paracetamol and haloperidol. He had, of course, already been placed on a water restriction regimen on account of suspected recurrence of psychogenic polydipsia.

Still on water restriction, he was returned to the general hospital from which he was initially referred. At this stage he was neither responding to his name nor to verbal commands, but he did respond to pain. However, within a few hours he was able to get out of bed and began wandering around; indeed, he became quite restless and had to be sedated with chlorpromazine. The serum sodium concentration rose steadily thereafter with continued water restriction (< 1.0 l/24 h), which was considerably less than hitherto, although much in excess of the < 0.5 l normally permitted a patient with severe water intoxication, e.g. from the syndrome of inappropriate ADH (SIADH) secretion. He was soon transferred back from the general hospital to the psychiatric hospital of origin, although the water restriction regimen was now made rather less severe as a compromise, in order to cause him the minimum of stress on account of his accustomed very high fluid intake.

This patient with psychogenic polydipsia of unusually severe degree was unable to effectively excrete the excessively high fluid load because the excretory capacity of the renal system had been exceeded. The normal kidney cannot excrete > 1.0 l/h, with the result that if fluid intake is very high the extracellular volume expands, thereby producing cerebral hydraemia (in which disorder there is inhibition of depolarization, which is itself the basis of nerve conduction).

Moreover, this patient's therapy included several drugs which could interfere with water balance (i.e. which could either compound or even partially alleviate the basic disorder). Paracetamol, for instance, can potentiate the action of antidiuretic hormone (ADH) on the distal renal tubule, phenytoin can suppress ADH release, and chlorpromazine is a phenothiazine which causes anticholinergic effects (i.e. the consequent dryness of the mouth could lead to increased fluid intake in an attempt to quench thirst). However, a definitive cause for this episode of psychogenic polydipsia was not established.

CASE 7

Clinical history

A 43-year-old man presented to his general practitioner; according to his wife he 'went to pieces' 2 weeks after his mother's death on 06.01.82. He became depressed and was put on tranquillizers, although they did not really help; in fact, he slowed down more and eventually became worse. Eight months later in September 1982 his wife suggested he might feel better if he had a holiday; accordingly they went to Spain for one week. However, it turned out to be the worst holiday they had ever had because he was ill all the time, was not able to eat and continued to be depressed, which was quite out of character because he was normally a vivacious and happy individual. He returned home to make an urgent appointment with his doctor who established a 5-month history of anorexia, weakness, nausea and loss of 4 stones in weight. On clinical examination, however, he appeared not to be unwell, but there was dark pigmentation in the mouth, of the palmar creases and on the chest. His blood pressure lying down was 100/70 mmHg, but on standing was 80/50 mmHg.

Laboratory investigations

Initially, on 23.09.82, the serum sodium concentration was 130 mmol/l (RR 135–147), the serum potassium 5.9 mmol/l (RR 3.5–5.0) and the serum urea 18 mmol/l (RR 2.6–6.5). The basal serum cortisol was 115 nmol/l (RR 221–773) at 09.00 h and the value 30 min after an intravenous injection of 250 µg tetracosactrin (Synacthen) in the tetracosactrin

(Synacthen) stimulation test (short procedure) was unchanged at 107 nmol/l. The plasma ACTH was elevated at 1907 ng/l (RR < 10–80). On 04.11.82 it was reported that adrenal antibodies were not detected.

Date	Serum sodium (mmol/l)	Serum potassium (mmol/l)	Serum urea (mmol/l)	Serum osmolality (mosmol/kg)	Serum LDH (IU/l)	Serum AST (IU/l)	Serum ALT (IU/l)
23.09.82	130	5.9	18.0	–	142	31	–
27.09.82	135	5.5	9.5	–	–	–	–
04.11.82	139	4.6	6.0	–	–	–	–
10.02.83	122	5.3	10.0	–	–	–	–
11.02.83	130	5.4	8.6	–	–	–	–
14.02.83	128	5.9	5.3	–	–	–	–
15.02.83	123	5.3	13.0	–	–	–	–
17.02.83	129	4.8	10.0	–	566	131	62
18.02.83	121	4.9	19.6	–	–	–	–
19.02.83	123	3.9	17.5	–	–	–	–
21.02.83	127	4.2	6.2	–	–	–	–
22.02.83	123	3.1	4.1	245	373	67	57
23.02.83	125	3.5	6.0	260	–	–	–
25.02.83	131	3.3	7.8	263	341	93	87
01.03.83	130	4.2	8.5	267	–	–	–
04.03.83	–	–	–	266	–	–	–
06.03.83	128	4.8	7.2	259	–	–	–

Analysis and comments

The lack of response in the tetracosactrin (Synacthen) stimulation test (short procedure), following the findings of a low serum sodium concentration, raised serum potassium and elevated serum urea, is typical of Addison's disease. Accordingly, parenteral hydrocortisone treatment was commenced without delay; later, cortisone acetate and fludrocortisone were substituted. He responded well and was allowed to return home.

However, about 3 months later, in January 1983, he again complained of anorexia and vomiting, but this time there was right-sided lower abdominal pain and flatulence. A markedly blood-stained stool precipitated admission to hospital; a mass was now palpable in the right iliac fossa. Ultrasound examination of the abdomen was unhelpful, but a barium follow-through examination showed an irregular terminal ileum and caecum, thought to be due to either a tumour or an abscess.

On 14.02.83 an exploratory laparotomy was performed, which revealed a mass arising in the caecum, also involving the terminal ileum. There were enlarged mesenteric lymph nodes, but the liver appeared normal. A right hemicolectomy was performed. On opening the resected specimen there was a yellowish-coloured submucosal tumour spreading through most of the wall of the caecum. Histologically, the tumour was reported to be a leiomyosarcoma of the caecum.

The initial post-operative recovery period was marred by an Addisonian crisis, caused by failure to administer increased steroids at a time of special need; there followed a brisk response to the increased parenteral steroid supplements. On 14.02.83, the day of the operation, the serum sodium concentration was recorded at 128 mmol/l and the serum potassium 5.9 mmol/l. On 17.02.83 the serum lactate dehydrogenase (LDH) was elevatated at 566 IU/l (RR 100–275) as also was the aspartate transaminase of 131 IU/l (RR 7–40) and alanine transaminase of 62 IU/l (RR 7–40); all three enzymes remained elevated thereafter.

However, on 22.02.83 (one week post-operatively) he was noted to be more depressed and lethargic with a varying degree of confusion. He had been becoming increasingly hyponatraemic and hypokalaemic during this week, in spite of continuing steroid therapy, and the serum osmolality was 245 mosmol/kg. He was diagnosed as having the syndrome of inappropriate ADH (SIADH) secretion. Water restriction partially improved, but did not entirely solve, the clinical and biochemical picture; the serum sodium concentration rose slowly over the next week and settled to around 130 mmol/l on 01.03.83; the urine sodium concentrations were inapproprately high for the low serum sodium values at this time.

On 04.03.83 the urine osmolality was 791 mosmol/kg in the presence of a serum osmolality of 266 mosmol/kg; the urine arginine vasopressin (AVP) level was 6.4 pmol/l which was reported to be inappropriately raised for the serum osmolality value.

On 05.03.83, 19 days after the operation, he became more confused, but without any significant change in either serum sodium concentration or urine osmolality. He developed grand mal epileptic fits and continued to be depressed. These symptoms were partially controlled by phenytoin sodium therapy. Nevertheless, his general condition deteriorated and he died on 07.03.83.

On his final admission to hospital his wife explained that the main cause of distress over the previous year had been his persistent depression. At first this appeared to be reactive, but in retrospect it had persisted longer and was of more severe degree than would normally be expected; moreover, it merged into the clinical expression of Addison's disease – and it is well known that the usual features of this disorder may occasionally be preceded by depression of up to 1–2 years duration. This state merged into the SIADH situation (perhaps because of the pain and stress following lower abdominal surgery), a typical expression of which is depression, confusion and slowness of mental processes. Moreover, neoplasia in its own right can, rarely, be preceded by up to 1–2 years of depression. Finally, subcortical metastases in the cerebrum, confirmed to be present at postmortem examination, could well be accompanied by 'flatness of mood' terminally, and could also be a reason for the SIADH syndrome. All this must be viewed against the background of a hitherto normally happy individual, who was often the 'life and soul' of the party, and who previously possessed on out-going personality. His wife said that instead of him continuing to be the dominant member of the household, he had become very submissive. Hence, a multiplicity of causes, sequentially and/or in varying combinations, could have accounted for the depressive symptoms of this patient.

Addison's disease is usually due to autoimmune disease of the adrenal cortex in Western countries. However, in this patient the test for serum adrenal antibodies was negative and it was subsequently found that he had a leiomyosarcoma of the caecum. It was postulated that he had developed the clinical expression of adrenocortical insufficiency on account of metastases in both the right and left adrenal cortex prior to clinical expression of the primary tumour. This, too, was confirmed at postmortem examination; the adrenal glands were almost entirely replaced by tumour. It is well known that a tumour of the caecum may present later than one in the descending colon because of the more fluid consistency of the bowel contents on that side. The elevated serum levels of LDH, AST and ALT were consistent with the hepatic secondary deposits which were present.

Water depletion

Clinical aspects

Water depletion (causing a hyperosmolar state) can be caused by reduction or cessation of H_2O intake for any reason, e.g. lack of available H_2O to drink, dysphagia, stupor/coma, or excessive loss in the urine as in diabetes insipidus, diabetes mellitus and chronic renal failure, where there has also been insufficient replacement of fluid. The occurrence of diarrhoea, vomiting or sweating may compound the situation. In the conscious patient, there is weight loss, thirst and dryness of the mouth. Dehydration is less overt than in sodium depletion on account of the greatest loss being from the intracellular compartment. As the condition progresses there is increasing lethargy, mental confusion, delirium, stupor and coma. At risk, in particular, are the elderly who have a lessened ability to accommodate to such changes; some patients lack thirst. In post-operative and incontinent elderly patients dehydration may be seen – with the consequence of confusion, secondary to inadequate fluid intake.

Biochemical basis

A steadily rising serum sodium, chloride and urea concentration leads to hyperosmolality which, in turn, leads to osmotic effects within the CNS; disturbance of electrical transmission is the outcome.

In diabetic ketoacidosis, non-ketotic hyperglycaemia and renal failure, where the molecules contributing to the hyperosmolar state are glucose and urea respectively, similar osmotic effects are produced within the CNS. The degree of consciousness in diabetic coma correlates with plasma osmolality, whereas in uraemia the relationship is less clear on account of the urea molecule possessing greater diffusibility; the implication is that the osmotic shrinkage of the brain is less. In uraemia and ketotic diabetic coma metabolic acidosis also contributes to the CNS disturbance.

However, commoner than H_2O depletion alone is the loss of H_2O and sodium together, in which case serum sodium concentration provides an index of the relative loss of each. Should there be very marked sodium depletion then hypovolaemia may lead to H_2O retention and hyponatraemia. Thus, serum sodium levels vary according to clinical circumstances – being low, normal or even elevated.

CASE 8

Clinical history

A 74-year-old lady was, at the request of her sister who lived with her, visited by the general practitioner. She had been unwell over the past week and was now 'flat' in mood, was somewhat confused, appeared vacant and was clearly withdrawn. There was a long-standing history of depression, but she was currently not receiving treatment for this. Accordingly, arrangements were made on 16.06.90 to admit her urgently to the local psychiatric hospital. However, whilst on her way there in the ambulance she had an epileptic fit, and was taken instead to the accident and emergency department of the local general hospital.

On further questioning the sister revealed that the patient was currently being treated with metronidazole for non-specific vaginitis, due to *Gardnerella vaginalis* infection. Shortly after therapy commenced she developed nausea, which was followed by persistent vomiting. She became unwell, was mentally withdrawn and started to be confused; over the last few days she had also been passing 'lots of water'. Current medication included temazepam 20 mg nocte and bendrofluazide 5 mg daily; the latter had only recently commenced, having been changed from Moduretic (comprising a mixture of amiloride hydrochloride and hydrochlorothiazide). Her past history included hysterectomy and partial thyroidectomy.

On clinical examination in hospital the patient responded sensibly to verbal commands, but much of the time she had a 'blank and vacant' appearance. She was seen to be dehydrated, emaciated and pale. Her pulse was 64/min and her blood pressure was 170/70 mmHg; the jugular venous pressure was not elevated. She was promptly admitted to the intensive care unit.

Laboratory investigations

Initially, on 16.06.90, there was gross electrolyte imbalance. Soon after admission the serum osmolality was found to be 250 mosmol/kg (RR 280–290), but the urine osmolality was inappropriately high at 510 mosmol/kg.

Date	Serum sodium (mmol/l)	Serum potassium (mmol/l)	Serum chloride (mmol/l)	Serum bicarbonate (mmol/l)	Serum urea (mmol/l)	Serum osmolality (mosmol/kg)
16.06.90	112	1.5	54	45.5	7.4	–
16.06.90	115	1.5	58	47.1	7.9	–
16.06.90	118	1.9	68	40.9	7.5	250
16.06.90	125	2.8	–	–	6.8	–
17.06.90	129	2.1	79	40.7	5.6	262
18.06.90	128	3.9	91	35.3	4.2	–
19.06.90	130	5.0	94	29.5	4.2	–
21.06.90	135	4.8	98	28.9	8.0	–

Analysis and comments

Management involved stopping the bendrofluazide therapy; fluids were also administered intravenously, together with potassium chloride and magnesium supplements. The metronidazole was also stopped and anti-emetics were given as and when required. The serum electrolyte results gradually improved over the next few days and eventually the infusions were withdrawn, at which time she was able to take fluids and food orally. On 22.06.90 she was eating well, and full clinical assessment showed that she was so much improved, both mentally and physically, that the psychiatric referral was cancelled. Accordingly, she was dis-charged home to be cared for by her sister, aided by the support of a social worker and the help of the community psychiatric nurse. No further appointment was made and she has remained mentally well ever since.

What at first appeared to be recurrence of a long-standing psychiatric problem was quickly revealed to be a consequence of gross electrolyte and water imbalance. Confirmation of this came in the form of a most satisfactory clinical response to correction of the imbalance. It is well rec-ognized that hyponatraemia can result from diuretic therapy, particularly in the elderly; hypokalaemia is a common accompaniment. Diuretic drugs can induce a lowering of circulating blood volume, following which (because of the potassium deficiency so often present) there may be an exaggerated response, via the baroreceptors in the region of the carotid bifurcation and in the left atrium, leading to excessive antidiuretic hor-mone (ADH) release. A rise of urinary osmolality and fall in serum osmo-lality follows. However, in this patient the problem was compounded by the administration of metronidazole, which induced nausea and vomiting;

the latter led to dehydration and metabolic alkalosis. Nausea and vomiting are also potent stimulants of ADH secretion, thereby producing powerful antidiuresis. The very recent exposure to metronidazole, in combination with the new diuretic, was the aetiology of this patient's serum electrolyte disturbance, secondary to which the psychiatric consequences ensued.

Hypernatraemia

Clinical aspects

There are a large number of causes of the hyperosmolar condition of hypernatraemia, amongst which are: (i) inadequate H_2O intake (e.g. as in coma, injury to the thalamic area of the brain, elderly confused patients, etc.), (ii) excess loss of H_2O through the skin (i.e. excessive sweating), gastrointestinal tract (i.e. vomiting and diarrhoea) and the renal tract (e.g. osmotic diuresis caused by glucose or urea) and (iii) excessive intake of sodium containing compounds (e.g. oral sodium chloride or bicarbonate). In essence, there are two types of hypernatraemia – those where dehydration is the cause and those where there has been sodium overload. Hypernatraemia does not necessarily equate with an excess of extracellular sodium. It is only when the serum sodium level rises to >160 mmol/l that hypernatraemic encephalopathy develops.

Clinical expression of severe hypernatraemia takes the form of thirst, lethargy, weakness, disorientation, confusion and, eventually, coma. In cases of lesser severity alteration in the level of consciousness may be the only sign.

Biochemical basis

It is hypertonicity within the extracellular space that causes the loss of cell H_2O in an attempt to re-create osmotic equilibrium between the two compartments. The result of these changes is that there is contraction of cell volume, which is basically responsible for the symptomatology referred to above, with haemorrhages secondary to shrinkage of cerebral tissue and consequent tension on the blood vessels. The latter can lead to mechanical tearing. Postmortem studies reveal both brain and meningeal haemorrhages and capillary thromboses.

CASE 9[82]

Clinical history

A 15-year-old girl had a 2-year history of depression and lethargy. For the last 6 months she had had failing concentration and memory, together with increasing visual difficulties. One week prior to being admitted to hospital for investigation she had found it awkward to walk on account of general weakness. She had only menstruated briefly at the age of 12 years. Nocturia had been present for 3 years, but there was no complaint of thirst. On examination she was noted to be drowsy and apathetic.

Laboratory investigations

Initially, the serum sodium concentration was elevated at 163 mmol/l (RR 135–147) and the serum urea was 3.3 mmol/l (RR 2.0–6.5). The urine specific gravity (SG) was never greater than 1.002 (i.e. disproportionately low compared with the serum sodium concentration). A diagnosis of diabetes insipidus had been made at this point and treatment with lysine vasopressin spray had been started, with marked improvement in the serum electrolytes. There was clinical suspicion of a hypothalamic disorder involving the optic chiasma. She was observed to be in fluid balance (i.e. the fluid intake equalled the urinary output; she was not clinically dehydrated).

	Serum sodium (mmol/l)	Serum osmolality (mosmol/kg)	Urine sodium (mmol/l)	Urine osmolality (mosmol/kg)	Urine SG
Initial findings	163	–	–	–	1.002
Preoperatively (10 days)	166	356	–	–	–
Preoperatively (7 days)	170	357	10	201	–
Rehydration	144	296	–	–	–
Excess vasopressin	124	255	–	–	–
Postoperatively (day 1)	–	–	–	–	1.018
Postoperatively (day 12)	160	332	–	–	–
Maximum serum osmolality with urine osmolality rising	–	370	–	396	–

Analysis and comments

Lumbar air encephalography showed an abnormality of the third ventricle and chiasmatic cistern. This suggested the possibility of an intrinsic tumour involving the hypothalamus and optic chiasma. A right frontal craniotomy and chiasmal exploration was performed, which revealed some pathological tissue around the posterior end of the optic chiasma; a biopsy was taken.

On the first day postoperatively she passed in excess of 8.0 l of urine; a diagnosis of diabetes insipidus was made and she was therefore treated with vasopressin. The result was that the urine SG promptly rose to 1.018. By the seventh day serum and urine electrolyte concentrations and osmolalities were within normal limits; moreover, the preoperative drowsiness and weakness had diminished. Five days later the serum osmolality rose again, to 332 mosmol/kg, and the serum sodium concentration was 160 mmol/l; increasing the vasopressin dose solved this. She was accordingly discharged from hospital 2 weeks later.

Regrettably her condition deteriorated and she died in status epilepticus 5 months later. The postmortem examination revealed the presence of a mass arising from the floor of the third ventricle, extending from the optic chiasma to the mammillary bodies, which it had replaced. The hypothalamus was compressed and infiltrated by the tissue. The paraventricular nuclei were infiltrated by tumour cells, as also were the supraoptic nuclei. Histologically the tumour was identified as a germinoma.

In the presence of a neurological disorder the possibility of the syndrome of hypothalamic adipsia/hypodipsia must be considered when there is hypernatraemia, absence of thirst, lethargy and apathy. Such patients are not overtly clinically dehydrated, presumably because there is pure water depletion which comes largely from the intracellular compartment. It has long been recognized that in the absence of dehydration, elevated serum sodium can be accounted for merely by re-setting of the 'osmostat', thus leading to release of ADH only when the serum osmolality reaches a higher than usual level. There is evidence for such a situation in this patient in that the urine osmolality achieved 396 mosmol/kg – but not until the serum osmolality had risen to 370 mosmol/kg.

CASE 10[83]

Clinical history

A 57-year-old lady was seen by her general practitioner on the evening of 25.02.74 because she had become disorientated and had developed diarrhoea; she was becoming increasingly delirious and mentally disturbed. The doctor examined her and made a clinical diagnosis of gastroenteritis, following which he gave, in order to sedate her, an injection of morphine. Her husband had explained that she was perfectly well up to this point, had eaten her evening meal and had enjoyed it in the normal way – but that it did include some peas. She then suddenly remembered the strict instructions given to her saying that she should not eat green vegetables on the evening before a special X-ray examination which was scheduled for the next day. Accordingly, she looked in her books at home to find out how she could make herself vomit; the advice given therein was to drink a solution of common salt.

On the following day the husband called the general practitioner again because by this time his wife was unconscious and was groaning. The diagnosis was now changed to that of bronchopneumonia and she was promptly admitted to hospital at 15.00 h on 26.02.74. Whilst in the accident and emergency department it was recorded that she was unconscious. It was felt that the differential diagnosis lay between an overdose of barbiturates (there were blisters, similar to those seen in such cases, on the inside surfaces of both knees and on the dorsum of the hand), meningitis and bronchopneumonia. The only past history obtained was that of a previous psychiatric illness and a nephrectomy operation just 1 year previously, on account of hydronephrosis.

Laboratory investigations

Initially, on admission, the serum sodium concentration was > 160 mmol/l (RR 135–147), and the serum chloride > 130 mmol/l (RR 95–107); the serum osmolality was 383 mosmol/kg (RR 280–290) and the bicarbonate was 14.8 mmol/l (RR 21–30).

Date	Serum sodium (mmol/l)	Serum potassium (mmol/l)	Serum chloride (mmol/l)	Serum bicarbonate (mmol/l)	Serum osmolality (mosmol/kg)	Serum urea (mmol/l)
26.02.74	> 160	3.1	> 130	14.8	383	9.3
26.02.74	> 160	2.8	> 130	12.0	369	10.3
26.02.74	145	3.4	122	10.0	350	9.0
27.02.74	136	3.1	106	20.5	324	7.6
27.02.74	137	3.8	107	16.0	296	5.6
28.02.74	130	4.2	97	23.0	270	6.0
08.03.74	132	4.2	94	28.0	–	8.1
22.03.74	137	3.6	96	25.0	–	7.0

Analysis and comments

Having identified the presence of an extremely severe degree of hyper-natraemia, the next step was to establish the cause. Accordingly, this was felt to be attributable to her known ingestion of strong salt solution, taken with the intention of inducing vomiting. Definitive therapy began 2.5 h after admission at 17.30 h, and comprised frusemide and dextrose given as quickly as possible by intravenous infusion. By 09.00 h on the following day the serum electrolytes were all within their reference ranges. However, generalized convulsions began during therapy and continued for 2 days, in spite of the high doses of antiepileptic compounds given intravenously. The convulsions ceased after 48 h and consciousness returned over the week. She was, however, left severely handicapped mentally, and spent much of the next 3 months clutching a doll. She was then referred to a local psychiatric hospital where she was cared for over the next 4 years, until she developed bronchopneumonia and died.

An oral overload of highly concentrated sodium chloride solution is rapidly absorbed in the intestine. Hence, the serum sodium and chloride concentrations rise rapidly, producing an acute hyperosmolar state as shown by the high serum osmolality values. There follows an osmotic shift of water from the intracellular compartment to the extracellular fluid (ECF).

Following rehydration of such a patient there would be a fall in tonicity of the ECF, creating a situation of relative hypertonicity intracellularly which, in turn, causes water to now enter the cells, leading to intracellular overhydration.

Should death occur in the acute stages, a postmortem examination would reveal bleeding within the brain and/or meninges, together with capillary thromboses caused by shearing stresses applied to the blood vessels when brain (and CSF) volumes change. The combination of brain shrinkage and intracranial blood vessel distension, in association with a rise of blood volume, may be the basis of subarachnoid haemorrhage and intraventricular haemorrhage in some instances.

In this patient there was, in the acute stages following salt ingestion, disorientation, delirium and mental confusion, at a time when serum electrolyte changes were occurring rapidly and when osmotic shifts would have been taking place. Subsequently, the cerebral damage which resulted was seen to have been permanent as indicated by the severe mental handicap that remained; proper cell functioning had clearly been severely impaired, this being secondary to changes in brain cell volume and tonicity.

VITAMIN DISORDERS[84]

Both fat soluble and water soluble vitamins, either in excess or deficiency, are indirectly implicated (by way of secondary biochemical changes) in mood alterations or frank psychiatric disorders; there may also, of course, be other accompanying clinical features. Vitamin D disorders will not be discussed in this section; it seems more convenient to include them under 'Mineral disorders', because the consequent changes in calcium metabolism underlie the mental features.

Vitamin B_1 (thiamine) deficiency[71,84]

Clinical aspects

Deficiency of vitamin B_1 is a problem in many elderly people, some of whom also express the deficiency following stress (e.g. caused by surgery or acute infection) in the form of confusion. The overt forms of vitamin B_1 deficiency comprise Wernicke's encephalopathy and Korsakoff's psychosis – as described below.

Wernicke's encephalopathy[71,84] is a cerebral form of thiamine deficiency presenting either acutely or unfolding rapidly over several days. It is most commonly seen in chronic alcoholics; these people rely on alcohol, rather than food, for their source of energy. They may be deficient in thiamine for several reasons (e.g. nutritional insufficiency, impaired gastrointestinal absorption of the vitamin, inability of the liver to store and utilize the vitamin because of the presence of cirrhosis and because of the high requirement for thiamine in the metabolism of alcohol). Apart from alcoholism the disorder may also be found in starvation, malnutrition, administration of inadequate parenteral nutrition in gastrointestinal problems and in cases of persistent vomiting.

There may be prodromal symptoms in the form of mild delirium, agitation, inability to sleep and hallucinations. The patient may become apathetic, be inattentive, sleepy, confused and disorientated; occasionally there may be progression to stupor and coma. Amnesia for new information may sometimes be found. In response to treatment with thiamine confusion may slowly improve over a few days or weeks, perhaps allowing any memory defect to come to light; the latter would take longer to improve. However, some patients may be left with a residual memory defect, i.e. Korsakoff's amnestic syndrome (Korsakoff's psychosis).

Neuropathological findings in acute cases of Wernicke's encephalopathy comprise petechial haemorrhages in and around the mammillary bodies, the floor and walls of the third ventricle, the aqueduct and floor of the fourth ventricle; the anterior nucleus of the thalamus may in some cases be similarly involved. Subacute cases show a lesser degree of involvement with the neurones being relatively unaffected; there is, however, capillary dilatation and proliferation in the same areas.

Korsakoff's psychosis[71,84] is characterized by defective ability to form new memories (anterograde amnesia), difficulty in recalling recent memories (retrograde amnesia), disorientation in both time and place and confabulation. Although immediate memory recall is excellent, just a few minutes later those memories will not be recalled. Judgement, however, remains intact.

In Korsakoff's psychosis the mammillary bodies are atrophied and display brown discoloration in those patients not responding to thiamine administration; there is, in addition, damage to the dorsal medial nucleus of the thalamus in those with defects of memory.

Biochemical basis

Thiamine, in the form of thiamine pyrophosphate (TPP), acts as coenzyme for certain enzyme reactions in the metabolism of carbohydrate and amino acids, e.g. the decarboxylation of pyruvate to acetyl CoA *via* pyruvate dehydrogenase (providing the connection between the anaerobic glycolytic pathway and Kreb's tricarboxylic acid cycle), the transketolase reaction (in the hexose monophosphate shunt), the decarboxylation of α-ketoglutarate to succinate *via* α-ketoglutarate dehydrogenase (in Kreb's cycle) and branched-chain α-ketoacid dehydrogenase. Cells deficient in thiamine are unable to utilize glucose aerobically; in this context the CNS in particular is in danger because of its absolute dependency on the delivery of glucose for energy needs. In addition to its role as coenzyme, thiamine and TPP may also function in maintaining neuronal membrane electrical activity. Defects in some of these biochemical pathways may underlie Wernicke's encephalopathy and Korsakoff's psychosis; some authorities regard the 'Wernicke–Korsakoff syndrome' as an entity.

CASE 11

Clinical history

A 73-year-old lady was admitted to hospital on 24.10.89 with chronic bronchitis and pneumonia. She had a long-standing history of chronic obstructive airways disease and had been receiving therapy with prednisolone, ipratropium bromide, salbutamol, beclomethasone dipropionate, aminophylline, metoclopramide hydrochloride, ranitidine, loperamide hydrochloride and Frumil (comprising a mixture of amiloride hydrochloride and frusemide). The day after admission she unexpectedly had a melaena stool and vomited 150 ml of blood. She had an urgent gastroscopy examination followed by an emergency laparotomy and blood transfusion. A large posterior gastric ulcer was found to be perforating into the pancreatic bed and transverse colon. A partial gastrectomy operation followed and she gradually improved over the next few weeks. Almost 2 weeks after the operation, on 05.12.89, it was commented that two major problems were present: the first was postoperative weight loss and the development of hypoalbuminaemia on

---

account of a long period without nutrition, and the second was that of recurrent diarrhoea.

On 16.02.90 she was re-admitted with upper abdominal pain (later extending over the whole abdomen), vomiting and clinical signs of peritonitis, for which she had a further laparotomy the following day. Dense adhesions of the small intestine and purulent fluid in the peritoneal cavity, oedema and inflammation of the retroperitoneal tissues were found. A faecal fistula, presumed to have come from an area of diverticular disease in the sigmoid colon, subsequently developed. After this had healed two more fistulae followed.

Despite the adverse circumstances of steroid dependency, basal chest infection and acute asthma, the patient made a slow but good recovery. However, the postoperative period was slowed by her unwillingness to eat and the onset of depression. She became more withdrawn as time progressed, refusing to communicate or answer questions, being unresponsive to instructions and commands, not moving her limbs spontaneously and, indeed, not making any sound. The nursing staff commented that she was slow in assisting or helping herself and that she was lethargic and 'doesn't speak'. All these features developed and progressed. Treatment with imipramine commenced on 29.03.90, but as improvement in depression may not occur during the first 2–4 weeks of treatment in many cases it was not expected that she would necessarily respond rapidly.

Laboratory investigations

Date	Serum sodium (mmol/l)	Serum urea (mmol/l)	Serum osmolality (mosmol/kg)	Serum total protein (g/l)	Serum albumin (g/l)	Serum AP (IU/l)
30.11.89	126	4.9	–	50	23	176
05.01.90	133	3.8	–	49	24	130
16.02.90	133	4.0	–	57	30	104
19.02.90	137	3.6	–	41	20	83
22.02.90	135	1.7	–	–	–	–
01.03.90	129	3.6	–	–	–	–
03.03.90	122	6.3	250	55	26	183
14.03.90	124	3.7	251	56	24	191
22.03.90	118	6.1	250	54	23	188
02.04.90	121	6.4	248	–	–	–

continued

Laboratory investigations continued

Date	Serum sodium (mmol/l)	Serum urea (mmol/l)	Serum osmolality (mosmol/kg)	Serum total protein (g/l)	Serum albumin (g/l)	Serum AP (IU/l)
04.04.90	118	7.0	247	60	28	216
08.04.90	121	5.8	250	–	–	–
11.04.90	129	5.8	262	51 ·	25	183
15.04.90	133	5.2	–	–	–	–
14.05.90	135	2.8	–	58	28	133
18.06.90	–	–	–	55	33	–
29.11.90	–	–	–	65	39	142
11.04.91	–	–	–	63	40	119

Analysis and comments

A detailed analysis of this patient's history and management was undertaken on 06.04.90, at which time it was very clear that her nutritional intake had been minimal/non-existent for a considerable period. She had, over this time, developed hypoalbuminaemia and hyponatraemia. However, of particular note was the observation that thiamine (vitamin B_1) had not been a component of her management regimen. It is known that absence of thiamine intake, as may occur in patients with severe gastrointestinal disorders, over a period of as little as 3 weeks, can begin to produce irritability, confusion and depression, all of which rapidly respond to vitamin replacement therapy. It was recognized, too, that she was generally malnourished and would require intensive total parenteral nutrition (TPN), but the specific effect of massive doses of thiamine alone was ascertained first.

The patient was given thiamine hydrochloride 300 mg orally on 06.04.90, followed by 100 mg orally daily commencing later that same day. Within 2–3 days there had been a dramatic improvement, with the first glimmer of response being noted on the morning after the first dose, at which time she was observed to be more talkative. The following day, on 08.04.90, she was reported to be a little brighter and better in general. On 09.04.90 the patient was 'a little brighter this morning and ate lunch by herself!'; the ability to eat her lunch unaided in any way was absolutely out of context with her declining state over the last few weeks. The TPN commenced on 11.04.90 and continued along with the jejunal feeding which started on 12.04.90; she progressively but slowly improved. With daily thiamine therapy, together with the nutritional regimen to which reference has already been made, the patient improved so much that it was possible for the clinical record of 26.04.90 to include the statement 'the difference is amazing'.

It was stated at the beginning of this case history that the patient was receiving nine drugs; some of these may well affect appetite, or cause deficiencies of specific nutrients. Prednisolone, for instance, may well induce vitamin C deficiency, as is certainly the case with prednisone. There is an inter-relationship between vitamin C and thiamine: vitamin C has been shown to have a thiamine-sparing effect. Of note in this context is the fact that polypharmacy, particularly in the elderly, must immediately alert one to the possibility of nutritional complications.

Vitamin B_{12} (cobalamin) deficiency[84]

Clinical aspects

Pernicious anaemia is a disease of insidious onset, with or without neuropsychiatric accompaniment; the latter could occur prior to the onset of anaemia. The mild depression and lassitude often present is not always recognized by the patient, but the marked feeling of well-being which develops within 24 h of the first therapeutic dose of intramuscular vitamin B_{12} brings with it realization that the patient had not felt as well as had been thought. There may also be progression to irritability, a tendency to paranoia and nocturnal confusion. The psychiatric presentation may indeed ante-date other features of the illness by up to 2 years. Progressive dementia may occur, although it is unusual in the absence of neurological signs; affective disorders, schizophrenia, disorientation and delirium have all been documented.

The cerebral pathology comprises progression from demyelination to axonal degeneration and neuronal death, by which stage the condition is no longer reversible with vitamin B_{12} therapy; there is very little gliosis or neuronal damage. An increased incidence of pernicious anaemia is found in hypothyroidism, hyperthyroidism, Addison's disease, hypoparathyroidism and vitiligo.

Biochemical basis

Vitamin B_{12} in the human is a co-factor for two different enzyme systems. Methylcobalamin serves as coenzyme to N^5-methyltetrahydrofolate homocysteine methyltransferase which donates its methyl group to homocysteine during methionine synthesis, tetrahydrofolate being regenerated at the same time. Another coenzyme, 5'-deoxyadenosylcobalamin, is involved in the methylmalonyl-CoA mutase reaction in which succinyl CoA is generated. The activity of both these enzymes is reduced when vitamin B_{12} is deficient. In consequence, there is lack of methionine formation (which not only serves as a substrate for protein synthesis, but also is a precursor for transmethylation reactions in, e.g. neurotransmitter, phospholipid and protein metabolism) and failure to convert methylmalonate to succinyl CoA (with increased urinary excretion of methylmalonic acid).

Folic acid deficiency[85]

Clinical aspects

Folate deficiency, induced by anticonvulsant therapy, is associated with mood change in children. There may be neuropsychiatric symptoms such as a fall of IQ, neurotic disturbance, depression, dementia and schizophrenic-like psychoses. Moreover, deficiency of folate (which could be drug induced), accompanied by depression and dementia, occurs in up to 30% of psychiatric in-patients and an even higher percentage of psychogeriatric patients.

Biochemical basis

It is probable that methylfolate exerts a modulatory role on neurotransmission.

Vitamin B_3 (niacin) deficiency[84]

Clinical aspects

Pellagra can result from nutritional deficiency of vitamin B_3 (as induced by alcoholism, the anorexia of other psychiatric states or unavailability of foods containing this vitamin) and can itself induce psychiatric symptoms. In addition, it can rarely be due to the carcinoid syndrome; tryptophan metabolism is deviated along the 5HT pathway instead of to niacin and NAD formation (which is normally the major route). Another rare cause is Hartnup disease; in this case there is defective intestinal and renal transport for certain amino acids (i.e. tryptophan, alanine, serine, threonine, valine, leucine, isoleucine, phenylalanine, tyrosine, glutamine, asparagine and histidine).

The classical concept of pellagra is of dermatitis, diarrhoea and dementia – with death as the ultimate consequence. Various mental changes are seen at different stages. In the early phase there is simply insomnia and fatigue. Later, the patient becomes irritable and nervous and there is anxiety with depression. As the encephalopathy proceeds the mental processes slow down and memory impairment becomes evident; then comes disorientation, confusion, confabulation, episodic violent outbursts, paranoia and delusions. Therapy with vitamin B_3 induces improvement, within hours or days, of many of the psychiatric symptoms – but the dementia is not reversible.

Biochemical basis

Niacin refers to nicotinic acid and its derivatives; as such it forms part of the diet, but it can also be formed from tryptophan (in which sense it is not a vitamin). Niacin is a component of NAD and NADP, both of which are necessary for many oxidation and reduction reactions of intermediary metabolism; profound NAD and NADP deficiency would be totally incompatible with life. The psychiatric manifestations of pellagra might involve diminished 5HT formation from tryptophan.

Vitamin B_6 (pyridoxine) responsiveness[84]

Clinical aspects

It is well established that administration of oral contraceptives can lead to depression in some women, a proportion of whom have demonstrable disturbance in tryptophan metabolism following an orally administered tryptophan load, although actual vitamin B_6 deficiency seems not to have been demonstrated. A return to the normal excretory pattern occurs after taking pyridoxine 20 mg t.d.s.

Biochemical basis

It is thought that the mechanism of action is by way of stimulating tryptophan pyrrolase, which is the rate-limiting enzyme in the kynurenine pathway. There is no evidence of vitamin B_6 deficiency in these women; it is clearly a pharmacological response rather than a nutritional deficiency.

Vitamin C deficiency

Clinical toxicity

There has been reference to a 'neurological triad' of psychological disturbance, hypochondriasis and depression as an early feature of vitamin C deficiency.

Biochemical basis

The above disturbance could possibly be related to the role of vitamin C in the synthesis of neurotransmitters.

Vitamin A toxicity

Clinical aspects

In chronic vitamin A toxicity, as would occur with continuous high dosage for 3 months or more, the patient develops mental features apart from other signs and symptoms. These include irritability, fatigue, anorexia, drowsiness, difficulty in concentration and a rise of intracranial pressure. A single massive dose of vitamin A rapidly causes (in addition to the the almost identical general effects that occur with chronic exposure) drowsiness, irritability, somnolence and headache; skin desquamation commences at any time over the next few days. In infants, vitamin A toxicity is indicated by elevated intracranial pressure, as shown by a bulging anterior fontanelle.

Biochemical basis

Some patients with hypervitaminosis A develop hypercalcaemia and elevation of serum alkaline phosphatase. Vitamin A toxicity is, however, a rare cause of hypercalcaemia. Hydrocortisone therapy in vitamin A toxicity (as also in hypervitaminosis D) can rapidly revert the serum calcium level to within the reference range. However, withdrawal of the vitamin is normally all that is required in managing the disorder.

MINERAL DISORDERS

Mental changes are present in a number of clinical disorders in which there are either deficiencies or excesses of various minerals.

Hypercalcaemia[69]

Clinical aspects

Elevation of serum calcium levels occurs in a number of clinical disorders, in any of which psychiatric manifestations can accompany the other biological features. Such disorders include primary hyperparathyroidism, carcinomatosis (involving the skeletal system), malignant neoplasms secreting hormonal factors, sarcoidosis, vitamin D toxicity, etc. The more severe psychiatric changes are seen only when the serum calcium is grossly raised, but depression is the most common manifestation seen at lesser degrees of elevation. There may be no other mood change than fatigue and lack of initiative, although depression and lack of energy feature highly in many instances; there can also be tension, irritability and anxiety. Confusion is typical of very high serum calcium levels and there can be mental slowing and impairment of memory. Occasionally there may be paranoia, mania or hallucinations. Stupor and coma are the consequences of untreated progressive hypercalcaemia.

Biochemical basis

Calcium plays a role in neural transmission, nerve excitability and secretion of neurotransmitters. Should extracellular calcium concentration rise then hyperpolarization occurs, in contrast to the increased neural excitability typical of lowered extracellular calcium. There seems to be some relationship in general between the level of serum calcium and symptoms. Lack of initiative and drive together with affective disorders occur at around 3.0–4.0 mmol/l, delirium and

organic encephalopathy at 4.0–4.75 mmol/l and stupor and coma at
>4.75 mmol/l. However, these values are somewhat variable, some
patients having relatively few, if any, symptoms at a level at which others are frankly unwell.

CASE 12

Clinical history

A 77-year-old man was admitted to hospital on 11.01.84 with a history of
being slightly muddled in his mind over the previous few months; he had, in
addition, been unsteady on his feet. He had also been constipated over
this period. His wife, on direct questioning, admitted that he had not been
fully well over this period and that over the previous 2 weeks he had
become increasingly confused, tending to stay in bed all day and refusing
his food. He had developed a cough, too, but there was no fever.

On clinical examination he was noted to be a pleasant, cooperative
man, who was slightly confused and mildly dehydrated; although fully
conscious he was disorientated. The only past history obtained was that
he suffered from osteoarthritis of the spine for which he was being prescribed ibuprofen.

Laboratory investigations

Initially, on 10.01.84, his serum sodium concentration was 142 mmol/l
(RR 135–145), serum potassium 4.1 mmol/l (RR 3.5–5.0), serum chloride 96 mmol/l (RR 95–105), serum bicarbonate 30.0 mmol/l (RR 24–32),
serum urea 17.6 mmol/l (RR 2.5–6.5) and the serum creatinine
366 μmol/l (RR 60–120). The serum alkaline phosphatase (AP) was 323
IU/l (RR 30–125), serum calcium 3.94 mmol/l (RR 2.12–2.63), serum
phosphate 1.64 mmol/l (RR 0.8–1.5) and the serum albumin 38 g/l (RR
35–50). The haemoglobin concentration was 11.9 g/dl, white cell count
10.3×10^9/l, platelets 170×10^9/l and the erythrocyte sedimentation rate
(ESR) 82 mm/h; the blood film was unremarkable. On 11.01.84 the
serum free thyroxine (FT_4) was 10.7 pmol/l (RR 9–28) and the serum
TSH 1.5 mU/l (RR <5.5); the blood glucose value was 4.8 mmol/l (RR
3.0–5.5). His urinary calcium excretion was 9.1 mmol/24 h (RR 2.5–7.5)
on 18.01.84, the urine volume being 2.2 l. The ESR on 19.01.84 was
40 mm/h. On 27.01.84 the serum parathyroid hormone (PTH) level was
75 ng/l (RR <120). On 17.02.84 the serum AP was 490 IU/l, with the
bone isoenzyme being elevated.

Date	Serum calcium (mmol/l)	Serum phosphate (mmol/l)	Serum albumin (g/l)	Serum AP (IU/l)	Serum urea (mmol/l)	Serum creatinine (μmol/l)
17.02.83	2.40	1.05	40	96	–	–
10.01.84	3.94	1.64	38	323	17.6	366
11.01.84	4.05	1.65	40	322	18.2	364
16.01.84	2.87	0.84	36	291	–	–
17.01.84	2.70	1.07	32	279	15.8	227
19.01.84	2.44	0.93	37	470	–	–
23.01.84	2.32	1.05	38	605	19.5	192
27.01.84	2.25	0.78	38	710	20.7	174
01.02.84	2.12	0.90	37	645	–	166
15.02.84	2.25	0.82	37	490	–	–
22.02.84	2.13	0.94	38	259	9.4	141
07.03.84	2.37	1.03	40	232	11.6	145
21.03.84	2.42	0.94	40	224	9.9	139
04.04.84	2.53	1.17	43	239	–	–
04.05.84	2.26	0.74	41	144	–	–
24.07.84	2.35	1.08	43	74	–	–
17.06.86	–	–	–	–	8.5	149

Analysis and comments

After admission to hospital on 11.01.84 with confusion (in the presence of hypercalcaemia) the patient was rehydrated and given frusemide as necessary; oral prednisolone was also started. His mental state had not changed by the following day, but on 13.01.84 he was clinically improved. Within 3 days he was fully alert and walking around reasonably well. This improvement coincided with a reduction in the serum calcium concentration from 4.05 mmol/l on 11.01.84 to 2.87 mmol/l on 16.01.84. He was, by this time, well orientated and his prednisolone dosage was reduced to 10 mg t.d.s. On 18.01.84 he was reported to be quite cheerful and on 01.02.84 he was so much better that the dose of prednisolone could be lowered to 5 mg/day.

Hypercalcaemia is a well recognized cause of confusion, depression, and irritability; eventually, semi-coma and even coma may occur, should the level rise further. The cause of the hypercalcaemia was, at the time, thought most likely to be of neoplastic origin. The serum AP continued to rise over the course of the following 3 weeks and he was found to have, on 11.01.84, an elevated right diaphragm. No focal lung lesion was seen on chest X-ray, although he was a known smoker.

Tests were arranged to exclude myelomatosis. None of them were supportive of this in that the serum protein electrophoresis only showed elevation of the α_1 and α_2 globulin fractions, and on 19.01.84 the urine Bence-Jones protein was negative. The sputum was examined cytologically for malignant cells, but only inflammatory cells were seen.

Theoretically, the possible causes of hypercalcaemia in this situation include metastatic deposits in bone (with the consequent release of calcium into the circulation) and ectopic production by a tumour (e.g. a bronchial carcinoma) of PTH, a PTH-like compound, prostaglandins – or of osteoclast-activating factor (OAF) – particularly in myelomatosis. However, primary hyperparathyroidism is common enough to be present incidentally during the course of any illness, thereby leading to confusion in the interpretation of laboratory results. In this disorder, as long as renal function is normal, the serum calcium is usually elevated (or at the upper end of the reference range) and the serum phosphate is usually decreased (or at the lower end of the reference range). A very high serum calcium of the order found in this patient is most likely to be a pointer to malignancy, especially if the serum phosphate is also raised. Moreover, the serum AP activity was rapidly rising, and this was thought to indicate a serious cause. However, later findings were that the level proceeded to fall again over the next 3–4 months (during which time he continued to receive prednisolone in decreasing amounts, eventually reaching 2.5 mg/day) and its significance became less certain. The patient maintained his improvement in that on 04.05.84 his mental processes were quite clear, his mobility was good and he had no more constipation. The cause of the hypercalcaemia which he had had 4 months previously was never established with certainty. Indeed, the patient survived almost another 4 years, suffering only from attacks of bronchospasm which he had had for many years; there was no further reference to the episode of hypercalcaemia. He died on 06.12.87.

Hypocalcaemia[69]

Clinical aspects

Hypocalcaemia is much less common than hypercalcaemia. Its causes include chronic renal failure, hypoalbuminaemia, pancreatitis, hypomagnesaemia and anticonvulsant therapy. In addition, there are the various parathyroid-related disorders – such as transient hypoparathyroidism (sometimes seen after a partial thyroidectomy operation), hypoparathyroidism (of hereditary, autoimmune and degenerative origin), and pseudo-hypoparathyroidism (in which the parathyroid glands function normally, but where the tissues are resistant to PTH).

In general, the symptoms comprise paraesthesiae of the extremities and circumoral areas, muscle cramps, laryngeal spasm and convulsions, being dependent upon severity of the hypocalcaemia and the rapidity of onset. In cases secondary to post-thyroidectomy an acute organic reaction may occur, with delirium. In those presentations of insidiously slow onset the patients often do not recognize their problems until a late stage (and even then not fully until the improvement following therapy has occurred). These patients have lassitude, tension, irritability, emotional lability, difficulty in concentrating, depression, and impaired intellect – sometimes there may even be a psychosis.

Biochemical basis

Calcium plays an important role in neurotransmission, nerve excitability and secretion of neurotransmitter substances. Increased neural excitability is to be expected when there is lowering of extracellular calcium, accounting for paraesthesiae, muscle spasms and convulsions.

Magnesium deficiency[69,86]

Clinical aspects

Magnesium deficiency produces lethargy, fatigue, decreased mentation and depression.

CASE 13

Clinical history

A 31-year-old lady presented to the rheumatology out-patients department on 27.02.89 with a story of pain and stiffness in the hands which was worse in the mornings. There was no joint inflammation, nor were there any rheumatoid nodules and there was no family history of inflammatory arthritis; joint stiffness rather than pain was the main complaint. She was investigated over the next few weeks but did not seem to fit any of the recognisable patterns of arthritis and she was sero-negative for rheumatoid factor. The symptoms persisted, together with myalgia and severe malaise; there were no other systemic features (i.e. there was no loss of weight and no fever).

On 17.11.90 a very detailed review of her history was undertaken in an attempt to solve the problem. She admitted that all her symptoms were non-specific and that none individually were major. Collectively, however, they were 'troublesome and a nuisance'. Previously she had been reluctant to itemise the vast array of complaints to anyone, as each on its own sounded to be so minor. She felt that it might appear that she too readily complained of trivia – indeed, those close to her had sometimes regarded them as being 'in the mind', and there had been some encouragement for her to join the 'Myalgic Encephalomyelitis Association'. Apart from pains in the thighs which caused her to rub them frequently, and which dated from her mid-teens, she was completely well until 2½ years before, i.e. May 1988. At that time she became aware of stiffness in the fingers, noticed spasms of the 4th and 5th digits and found that sometimes her fingers would not open properly, particularly if she had been at rest for some time. There was also pain in the muscles generally, but never in a constant place, always moving around and mainly in the thighs and upper arms; the nature of the pain changed from time to time, varying from a dull pain to a stabbing sensation, sometimes prolonged, sometimes transient and 'hard to explain, really'. Tiredness was present, quite marked at times, and she now lacked the energy to which she had, previously, been accustomed; she was no longer able to work full-time as a hospital nurse because she was feeling somewhat despondent on account of the stress of her work.

In May 1989, one year after the onset of symptoms, she felt that all these feelings were becoming an integral part of her. Nevertheless, although accustomed to regular holidays abroad, she began to find that she no longer reacted well to flying; she was dizzy and 'everything seemed to be moving'. This puzzled her because she had never had such problems before. Shortly afterwards, whilst donating blood (which she had done regularly for many years) she fainted for the first time. She decided to leave her job as a hospital nurse and remained off-work for 4 months; however, to her surprise she felt no better at the end of this rest period. She continued to lack energy, was tired and the muscle pain persisted.

In November 1989 further problems developed. A rash had appeared over the abdomen creeping up the sides of the chest, it became itchy and there were spots. It troubled her on three or four occasions, slight pain being a feature. One knee swelled up for 2 days, for no apparent reason – but in a strange way it was a relief to her – because she could now show her doctor something tangible rather than merely recount a list of unproved symptoms.

Around May 1990 the sensation of pins and needles, already present for several months, became more marked and was noted to involve both arms and legs, particularly when sitting or lying in an awkward position; there were accompanying twitches and jerks of the muscles. There was also stiffness of the jaw when eating. A very mild form of pain in the knees also occurred. Some loss of strength was then observed to involve the arms, particularly during bed-making; she was now unable to hold her arms up as long as she should. There was, therefore, less stamina and she began to awaken with cramps in the calves of her legs. Vacuuming her carpets became a major and onerous task.

In August 1990 she had a 2-day episode of slight chest pain; some months later this recurred whilst vacuuming. The only long-term problem, revealed on direct questioning, was that mild 'hypoglycaemic attacks' had been occurring periodically for many years; these feelings of 'sweatiness and shakiness' had been relieved by eating small quantities of food more often. The attacks occurred at random intervals, but not after fasting or in the mornings; they did, however, bear some relationship to drinking alcohol.

There had been visits to a consultant gynaecologist since February 1990 on account of primary infertility. Her menses were essentially irregular, except for between 17 and 27 years of age during which time she was on the contraceptive pill. Her cycle was variable in length from 22–34 days and the bleeding was normally of 5 days duration. It was considered likely that she did not ovulate every month. In view of the poor quality of the cervical mucus found on two occasions therapy with ethinyl-oestradiol (20 µg/day on days 11 to 15 of the menstrual cycle) was commenced on 12.12.90, the aim being to increase the amount of cervical mucus. She was also given cyclofenil (200 mg b.d. on days 3 to 12 of the menstrual cycle) which is sometimes used in the therapy of anovulatory infertility where there is dysfunction of the hypothalamo–pituitary–ovarian axis. A significant improvement occurred in that her cervical mucus became much clearer. Both drugs were stopped, however, after it was found that serum activities of aspartate transaminase (AST), alanine transaminase (ALT), lactate dehydrogenase (LDH) and alkaline phosphatase (AP) were rising (although the rises were only slight they were significantly over and above her 'normal levels'); the highest recorded values were as follows: serum AST 249 IU/l (RR 7–40), serum ALT 345 IU/l (RR 7–40), serum LDH 223 IU/l (RR 90–180) and serum AP 22 IU/l (RR 30–125). Following the cessation of therapy on 28.03.91 all these enzyme activities began to fall after a few days.

Laboratory investigations

Date	Serum calcium (mmol/l)	Serum phosphate (mmol/l)	Serum albumin (g/l)	Serum AP (IU/l)	Serum PTH (ng/l)	Serum AST (IU/l)	Serum ALT (IU/l)	Serum LDH (IU/l)
27.02.89	–	–	47	14	–	30	17	144
13.11.89	2.27	1.45	42	14	–	23	13	141
12.02.90	2.26	1.27	42	13	–	26	14	133
30.08.90	2.13	1.58	40	14	21	30	17	145
17.11.90	2.23	1.32	41	12	15	–	–	–
08.03.91	2.29	1.59	39	22	10	103	185	150
26.03.91	2.44	1.54	44	20	–	249	345	223
03.04.91	2.27	1.28	41	20	–	147	224	172
09.05.91	2.18	1.30	42	12	–	51	41	135
17.05.91	2.30	–	42	–	–	–	–	–
17.06.91	2.15	–	42	–	16	–	–	–
24.06.91	2.33	1.13	40	13	–	28	18	115
24.09.91	2.36	1.36	41	10	–	22	15	120
25.11.91	2.27	1.35	39	13	–	22	14	111

Initially, on 27.02.89, the serum AP activity was 14 IU/l (RR 30–125); subsequently, the serum calcium level was found to be persistently towards the lower end of the reference range, being 2.27 mmol/l (RR 2.12–2.63) and the serum phosphate was persistently towards or above the upper end of the reference range, being 1.45 mmol/l (RR 0.8–1.5). The serum parathyroid hormone (PTH) level was low at 21 ng/l on 30.08.90 (RR 10–65). The phosphate excretion indices test was performed on 14.11.90, producing the following results: creatinine clearance 88 and 87 ml/min (RR 97–127), phosphate clearance (PC) 5.7 and 6.7 ml/min (RR 4–16), phosphate excretion ratio (PER) 0.06 and 0.08 (RR <0.15), phosphate excretion index (PEI) –0.11 and –0.09 (RR –0.09 to +0.09) and tubular reabsorption of phosphate (TRP) 111% and 109% (RR 84–95). On 19.11.90 the autoimmune profile was assessed; antinuclear antibodies (ANA) were negative, gastric parietal cells, mitochondria, smooth muscle, thyroglobulin, thyroid microsomes, gonadal steroid-producing cells and adrenal cortex, but positive to reticulin (titre of 1:20). The rheumatoid arthritis (RA) haemagglutination test was positive, too (titre of 1:80). The HEp-2 cell test for ANA was positive (speckled) and the parathyroid antibodies were also positive. On 17.11.90 the serum 25-hydroxycholecalciferol level was 14.4 µg/l (RR 3–30), the urine calcium on 19.11.90 was 5.5 mmol/24 h (RR 2.5–7.5) and the urine phosphate 21.6 mmol/24 h (RR varies with the dietary intake). The serum magnesium level was 0.82 mmol/l (RR 0.65–1.0).

On 14.01.91 an X-ray examination of the skull revealed no significant abnormality, with the pituitary fossa being of normal size. No intracranial calcification was seen.

Analysis and comments

This patient had a serum calcium concentration consistently towards the lower end of the reference range, and a serum phosphate consistently towards or above the upper end of the reference range. It is notable that the serum AP activity has always been low over the period of observation; the only time it increased at all (yet still remaining within its pathologically low range) was when she reacted to the drug regimen prescribed for her gynaecological disorder. It was most likely to have been the hepatic isoenzyme that was increased, and not the bone fraction in this instance. In the presence of a low (or low in the reference range) serum calcium and raised (or high in the reference range) serum phosphate, and in the absence of chronic renal failure, the implication is that the parathyroid glands are unable to secrete sufficient PTH to correct the situation, meaning that the very best performance they can achieve is not very good. Such findings are consistent with a diagnosis of primary hypoparathyroidism; furthermore, this is supported by the low in the reference range PC, the low PEI and the raised TRP. There is clearly only partial hypoparathyroidism here, otherwise the serum calcium value would be very much lower and the symptoms much more severe. The nature of the hypoparathyroidism is the next problem to be determined, and in this context it is seen that the patient was positive for serum antibodies to the parathyroid glands. Moreover, on examination of other members of her family, it was later found that parathyroid antibodies were also present in the serum of her mother, her father, her brother and her sister.

In November 1990 she was reassured, from the point of view of the muscle pains and tiredness, that there was nothing seriously wrong with her and that a large part of her symptomatology could be accounted for by underactivity of the parathyroid glands; accordingly, she was told that the previously considered diagnoses of myalgic encephalomyelitis, fibromyalgia and early inflammatory polyarthritis were no longer tenable. The stress of all the previous uncertainty was relieved as soon as she knew there was something tangible to satisfactorily account for her symptoms. She described her feelings at this time more as 'well-being' than true clinical improvement; indeed, she continued with the same clinical symptoms as before. However, on 21.02.91 treatment with alfacalcidol (1-α-hydroxycholecalciferol) was started at a dose of 1 µg/day.

On 16.05.91 tiredness still remained a feature, but the irritation and dryness of the skin (which commenced 2 weeks after the start of oestrogen therapy, and which was worse at around the time when the hepatic enzymes were elevated) was beginning to lessen. She was now beginning to experience progressive improvement generally, the 1-α-hydroxy-cholecalciferol having been taken for just over 3 months. By 17.06.91 the muscle pains had markedly decreased, and by 01.07.91 she was further improved, being less tired and complaining very little of muscle aching. On 29.07.91 there was no muscle pain at all. On 07.10.91 she was noted to be very well with only occasional twinges of muscle pain, although tiredness was still sometimes present at the end of the day; however, there was no marked accompanying change in serum levels of calcium and phosphate.

A high incidence of psychiatric features is noted to occur in patients with hypoparathyroidism, even higher in the more slowly developing idiopathic type than in those cases of rapid origin (e.g. post-thyroidectomy). In the latter group there tends to be, in those patients who do have such a response, an acute organic reaction in which delirium features. In those cases where the onset is insidious there tends to be emotional lability, difficulty with concentration and some impairment of intellectual function. Attention has been drawn to the features of partial hypoparathyroidism; these include tension, anxiety, attacks of panic, depression and lassitude.

Biochemical basis

Magnesium is an essential component of many enzyme systems; it is vital not only for cell membrane permeability, neuromuscular excitability, and muscular contraction, but also for protein, nucleic acid and fat synthesis.

Iron deficiency[87–89]

Clinical aspects

Even mild iron deficiency can lead to subtle behavioural changes with diminution of work performance, listlessness, fatigue and pica; all are rapidly reversible following correction of the iron deficiency state. In children with iron deficiency there may be impairment of learning ability, which is often irreversible; the degree of reversibility depends on the severity of iron deficiency and the age of the child. A study in which iron supplements were given to iron-deficient Asian children produced a good response mentally. Pica is an abnormal desire to eat strange substances or certain foods (e.g. carrots, tomatoes, vegetables, etc.) in excess; items that may be eaten include ice cubes (pagophagia), clay (geophagia), cornstarch (amylophagia), burnt match sticks (cautopyrophagia), coal, earth, soap and flakes of lead-containing paint as from an old cot (with the well-recognized danger of developing lead poisoning, particularly in children). Many of the items are crisp and crunchy – but even soft toilet paper may be the 'obsession'. Clearly, such patients do not go to their general practitioners complaining of eating coal and carrots – the story needs to be skilfully and patiently extracted from them; indeed, the true history may never be divulged, except reluctantly and by some strange chance.

Biochemical basis

Depletion of iron-containing enzymes and cofactors in tissue metabolism may be important in the development of these symptoms. As a component of haemoglobin, iron possesses a vital role in the transport of oxygen in the blood. Iron is also a component of MAO, an enzyme that plays a central role in the production of several neurotransmitters, namely DA, NA, adrenaline and 5HT. There is evidence that iron is essential for normal development and functioning of dopaminergic neurones, and it may be that deficiency of iron in early life could cause permanent damage to this system; animal experiments have revealed that rats with low iron content had fewer D_2 receptors. Iron is distributed unevenly in the brain, but it does seem to be found in relation to those neurones producing the inhibitory neurotransmitter GABA. Low levels of iron are thought either to interfere with GABA degradation or to impair normal performance of dopaminergic neurones.

Lead poisoning[74,86,89]

Clinical aspects

Inorganic lead salts can cause lead poisoning *via* ingestion or inhalation; pica (eating lead-containing paint chips) is often the basis in infants and children in particular and this, in turn, is often secondary to iron deficiency. A subclinical form of plumbism, with none of the general symptoms, can later present clinically with irreversible mental retardation when the growing brain is exposed to high amounts of lead; the consequences are failure of language development, disorders of cognitive function and abnormalities of behaviour. In children, mental changes occur if the condition is of sufficient severity, toxicity being indicated by irritability, hyperactivity, lethargy, convulsions and coma; cerebral oedema is an important factor in development of the encephalopathy. In the adult, there may be memory loss, together with other CNS signs; however, it is unusual for encephalopathy to develop at this time of life, except following exposure to tetraethyl lead when convulsions and confusion may occur.

Biochemical basis

Lead poisons enzyme systems by binding to disulphide groups. When present in high concentration there is denaturation of intracellular proteins following interference with their tertiary structures. Cell death with tissue inflammation follows. Blood lead levels are elevated.

Mercury poisoning[74,89]

Clinical aspects

Mercury poisoning can be acute or chronic; there can be inhalation of vapour or ingestion of inorganic or organic mercury; not all modes have a psychiatric accompaniment. Acute metallic mercury toxicity causes increased excitability. Chronic mercury vapour poisoning leads to lassitude and anorexia initially, but later there is mercurial erethism, characterized by timidity, emotional lability, excitability, loss of memory, insomnia, delirium, suicidal tendencies and a psychosis. It was erethism that once accounted for the problems encountered by felt hat makers who inhaled the hot mercuric nitrate that they used in making the felt – and hence the origin of the phrase 'as mad as a hatter'. Chronic inorganic mercury poisoning is the basis of acrodynia (pink disease) in children who typically develop irritability as part of the clinical presentation; it used to follow exposure to mercury-containing teething powder, ointments and medicaments. Acute and chronic organic mercury toxicity cannot easily be distinguished; postnatally, apart from other CNS involvement, there is memory loss, erethism, stupor and coma.

Biochemical basis

Biochemically, mercury poisons enzymes, having particular affinity for thiol groups.

Manganese toxicity[74,86,90]

Clinical aspects

Miners who have inhaled manganese dust over many months develop, in addition to extrapyramidal features, irritability, euphoria and emotional instability, followed by onset of lethargy, apathy and somnolence.

Biochemical basis

Manganese is a trace element which serves as an enzyme activator and is also a component of metalloenzymes.

Zinc deficiency[85,90]

Clinical aspects

In rare cases of zinc deficiency, apart from other clinical manifestations (such as skin lesions), mental apathy or depression is prominent.

Biochemical basis

Zinc is an intrinsic part of many metalloenzymes; it is essential for protein, DNA and RNA synthesis.

Thallium poisoning[74,89]

Clinical aspects

Acute poisoning will rapidly produce delirium. Subacute poisoning will lead to confusion, hallucinations, sleep disorders, convulsions, psychosis and dementia. After chronic thallium exposure there may be residual memory loss.

Biochemical basis

Thallium binds strongly to sulphydryl groups which are often present in enzyme systems, thus interfering with their functions; it also enters cells in exchange for potassium.

Selenium toxicity[90]

Clinical aspects

Excessive exposure to selenium fumes leads to apathy, lassitude, nervousness and depression, although these symptoms soon disappear following vacation of the area. Ingestion may cause fatigue and emotional lability.

Biochemical basis

Selenium is an antioxidant and as such is involved in the function of glutathione peroxidase.

Vanadium toxicity[86]

Clinical aspects

Lassitude and depression have been described in cases of vanadium poisoning; this information emanates mainly from the chemical manufacturing industry.

Biochemical basis

Inhibition of Na^+/K^+-ATPase which, in turn, inhibits the sodium pump results from vanadate (the pentavalent ion of vanadium) exposure.

Rubidium toxicity[86]

Clinical aspects

There is evidence for rubidium having an antidepressant effect; indeed, it is just over 100 years since the first report of subjective well-being was noted in a group of patients with cardiac disorders treated in this way.

Biochemical basis

Rubidium decreases ATPase activity and interferes with sodium binding; it also leads to increased NA turnover.

INHERITED METABOLIC DISORDERS[91,92]

Those inherited disorders referred to here are ones that do not necessarily present in infancy or childhood, but may be clinically expressed only during adolescence or in adult life. In general, they are rare, chronic disorders, which display insidious progression, although porphyria would be more correctly regarded as being intermittent.

Acute intermittent porphyria (AIP)[93]

Clinical aspects

AIP is a rare inborn error of metabolism of autosomal dominant inheritance; it is the most severe of the porphyric group of disorders, displaying a very variable degree of expression. Clinical presentation, commencing at puberty or later, assumes the form of recurrent attacks, each lasting from a few days up to a few months duration, and involving a multiplicity of neuropsychiatric features. Classically, there is acute abdominal pain on account of an autonomic neuropathy, often misdiagnosed as appendicitis. The psychiatric symptoms are often, but not necessarily present at the same time – although they may, in some cases, be dominant. Disorientation, confusion, delirium, coma and convulsions are the extreme manifestations, but restlessness, emotional lability, histrionic behaviour, severe depression and emotional instability may be observed. Psychiatric disorders resembling schizophrenia and paranoid reactions are well recognized. As regards the general personality it has been claimed that emotional instability and functional disturbances are typical.

Biochemical basis

Biochemically, there is reduced porphobilinogen (PBG) deaminase activity, with elevation of δ-aminolevulinic acid (δ-ALA) and PBG in the urine in attacks. Experimentally, it has been shown in animals that δ-ALA produces behavioural and biochemical effects; another suggestion has been that it serves as an inhibitor of GABA release from inhibitory nerve endings. However, the neurological features might also be related to intracellular haem deficiency, the biosynthesis of which is retarded when PBG deaminase is depressed. Probably less than one in three of all individuals showing the enzyme deficiency ever have symptoms of AIP. Such symptoms can be provoked by certain drugs (e.g. barbiturates, alcohol, anticonvulsants, etc.), hormones (e.g. oestrogens, oral contraceptives, etc.), other agents and circumstances (e.g. starvation, infections, etc.); emotional stress does not seem to be a precipitant. Furthermore, other mechanisms may also be implicated in the genesis of the psychiatric state (e.g. development of the SIADH syndrome); features of the latter disorder, superimposed upon the other metabolic disturbances, may create a complex situation.

CASE 14

Clinical history

A 22-year-old lady, with a history of anorexia nervosa of several years standing, starved herself for 2 days prior to going to a party at which she imbibed alcohol. She returned home after developing abdominal pain at 23.00 h on 15.10.84. The pain began in the lower central abdomen and worsened as it moved towards the right iliac fossa over a period of several hours. The general practitioner was called and arrangements were made to admit her to hospital. She felt nauseated, but there had been no vomiting. She had never had pain of this severity before. On clinical examination she was found to be tender over the whole of the abdomen, but more so on the right side; there was guarding with rigidity in the right iliac fossa. A confident diagnosis of appendicitis was made and she was taken to theatre without delay. At operation, however, the appendix was not inflamed, but there was increased non-haemosiderin pigmentation within the macrophages on histological examination. It was regarded that this indicated a condition analogous to melanosis coli, with implications relating to constipation and the use of purgatives. In this context it should be re-iterated that she had anorexia nervosa and that she did admit to taking laxatives 'at times'. At operation the ovaries appeared normal.

The following day the patient still complained of pain in the lower abdomen; an entry in the case notes also recorded the occurrence of pain in the right loin, frequency of urination, pyrexia and frank haematuria. The pain was severe and persistent, causing many requests for medical attention; the patient was behaving somewhat 'hysterically' according to some sources. 'Asked to see the patient again!' was inserted in the case notes several times, the overall impression being that the abdominal pain was much exaggerated. She was tender all over the abdomen, describing the feeling 'as though something is scraping my inside out, terrible!' and saying that the pain was 'like before the operation'. She became flushed with a temperature of 37.5 °C on 18.10.84. The results of the urine examination, performed by a nurse, were recorded in the case notes indicating both bilirubin and urobilinogen to be present. In spite of medication, the bowels had not been open for several days since the day of operation.

On 20.10.84 the patient was reported by another patient to have had a fit; she was found by the nurses to be drooling and drowsy. Shortly afterwards another fit was witnessed, this time by the nursing staff; her teeth were tightly clenched and there was a tonic and clonic phase, in addition to foaming at the mouth and cyanosis. There had been no past history of epilepsy. Several more grand mal fits occurred over the next few days. Following these she developed tachycardia, labile hypertension and urinary retention. She was disorientated and confused at times. She began to improve a few days later, had no more epileptic fits and became more alert and cooperative; she lost her recent confusion, disorientation and drowsiness and her bowels started to work again. Prior to discharge she complained of burning sensations which were at times severe, affecting mostly the upper thighs, around the shoulders and down the arms; all these improved before leaving hospital.

Laboratory investigations

The possibility of porphyria was first thought of on 21.10.84 when urine studies were requested. On 22.10.84 it was revealed that urinary porphobilinogen (PBG) was strongly positive and that porphyrins were also present.

Date	Serum sodium (mmol/l)	Serum potassium (mmol/l)	Serum chloride (mmol/l)	Serum bicarbonate (mmol/l)	Serum urea (mmol/l)
17.10.84	138	4.4	–	28.0	7.5
20.10.84	131	2.9	90	22.9	6.6
22.10.84	123	4.1	–	–	7.1
22.10.84	120	4.3	–	–	7.1
23.10.84	127	4.2	–	–	6.8
25.10.84	136	3.7	98	30.9	4.3
30.10.84	136	4.0	–	25.0	4.0
21.10.85	140	3.9	108	26.8	7.6
23.08.87	141	3.8	–	25.0	7.2
26.08.87	139	4.0	–	29.0	7.1
03.10.87	140	4.4	–	25.0	7.8
08.10.87	132	3.4	–	29.0	7.2
09.10.87	127	3.4	88	26.0	5.0
19.01.88	136	3.5	–	26.0	5.7
21.01.88	137	4.1	–	31.0	5.0
22.01.88	142	4.7	–	32.0	6.8

continued

Continued

Date	Serum sodium (mmol/l)	Serum potassium (mmol/l)	Serum chloride (mmol/l)	Serum bicarbonate (mmol/l)	Serum urea (mmol/l)
03.03.88	139	3.3	105	24.0	5.8
08.03.88	128	3.9	–	26.0	9.0
14.03.88	137	4.5	–	22.0	11.0
15.04.88	142	3.7	100	33.2	7.0
02.09.88	143	3.7	107	27.2	6.5
04.09.88	134	4.4	100	29.8	4.0
16.09.88	140	3.7	102	27.8	6.8
18.09.88	140	3.5	102	30.0	10.4
03.12.88	142	3.1	98	35.6	10.4
07.12.88	143	3.9	100	33.4	6.4
17.12.88	139	3.1	95	26.4	9.6
03.01.89	137	4.3	103	25.0	10.0
12.01.89	142	4.7	110	17.6	11.5
04.05.89	143	3.2	100	29.4	8.6
08.05.89	143	4.1	101	32.8	7.0
11.05.89	139	3.9	102	25.3	4.6
27.05.89	143	3.3	103	26.1	7.5
02.06.89	138	3.4	89	39.5	9.3
22.12.89	141	3.0	98	28.4	7.9
12.02.90	139	3.2	93	32.7	8.5
28.02.90	138	4.1	97	29.9	6.2
02.03.90	141	4.2	106	25.7	4.4
13.07.90	142	3.3	97	23.8	5.8
18.07.90	142	3.9	99	30.7	8.4

Analysis and comments

Subsequently, this patient had five further attacks of abdominal pain over the next 4 years, with the frequency increasing markedly thereafter to approximately five attacks per year. Every admission latterly, each with severe pain, has necessitated pethidine treatment in increasing amounts; moreover, each hospital admission has become longer in duration as time has advanced.

It is important to avoid hypoglycaemia in a patient with acute intermittent porphyria as this may precipitate an attack. Hence, the history of anorexia nervosa is important here, because a low carbohydrate intake is typical of the disorder. Starvation for 2 days prior to a party, and intake of alcohol, are both potential precipitants of a porphyric attack in an individual genetically predisposed. The final insult in this case was when thiopentone anaesthesia was given; this is a well recognized and powerful provocative agent in this context. It is no surprise, therefore, that she suffered continuous and severe pain after the operation. The patient is also reported to have had frank haematuria on the first day postoperatively. In retrospect, this was almost certainly the port-wine coloured urine of an attack of acute intermittent porphyria. The urine sample was never sent to the laboratory for analysis, however, and on the ward was clearly not examined closely enough. The 'orange' coloured urine noted a few days later was examined by a junior nurse; in her inexperience she mis-read the Multistix (Ames Division, Miles Laboratories Ltd.) test on the ward as positive for bilirubin and urobilinogen. Subsequent analysis of the same sample of urine a few days later in the laboratory confirmed that the colour change did not equate in any way with her conclusion.

The falling serum sodium concentration postoperatively occurred at about the same time as the epileptic fit. The syndrome of inappropriate ADH (SIADH) secretion is well recognized to occur during the course of acute intermittent porphyria, but is a rare phenomenon. The sensory neuropathic changes which this patient complained of before she left hospital may also be a feature of porphyria. Her genetic background is unknown as she was an adopted child.

It is of special note that metabolic alkalosis, sometimes accompanied by hypokalaemia, was a recurring feature in the period from October 1987 to July 1990, representative serum values for each of her admissions being included in the list of laboratory investigations. It is likely that vomiting was the cause; it could be that this was intentional (i.e. an integral component of the anorexia nervosa) or that it was done with the more subtle intention of creating the 'spin-off' complication of a porphyric attack, the gene for which disease she had by chance inherited, and which she might possibly have learned to manipulate in order to create a situation, if and whenever she so desired, with the aim of obtaining pethidine – for which she was rapidly developing a need.

Metachromatic leucodystrophy[71,91]

Clinical aspects

This disorder of autosomal recessive inheritance normally presents in childhood, but one in four cases present in adult life during the second to fifth decade; there is a male:female ratio of two to one. In addition to the dominant psychiatric aspects, there are also neurological features. Initially, there may be a falling off of intellectual performance at school or college, with forgetfulness and irrational behaviour appearing; emotional difficulties, suspiciousness, delusions and general personality problems also emerge. In adults the initial presentation may be in the form of a psychosis and dementia. Over the years the psychiatric state gradually deteriorates, with dementia being the end result.

Biochemical basis

The biochemical basis of this lysosomal storage disease is deficiency of arylsulphatase A (cerebroside sulphatase), leading to accumulation of cerebroside sulphates (galactosyl sulphatide) in Schwann cells, the myelin sheath and in other parts of the body; as a result there is an increase in urinary sulphatide and presence of metachromatic material in the urine. Neuropathologically, there is demyelination.

Adrenoleucodystrophy (X-linked Schilder's disease)[71]

Clinical aspects

This slowly progressive disorder presents with both Addison's disease and/or cerebral involvement. There is intellectual deterioration with dementia ultimately. Although adrenal corticoid therapy improves the Addison's disease, it does not influence the cerebral component of the illness. There are several other leucodystrophies apart from this particular condition. They include metachromatic leucodystrophy, globoid cell leucodystrophy, Pelizaeus–Merzbacher disease and Canavan's disease.

Biochemical basis

There is elevation of urinary C_{22}–C_{26} fatty acids. Demyelination is widespread in the brain. This disorder is one of several in which there is diffuse disintegration of the cerebral white matter, the cell bodies being relatively spared.

Adult G_{M2}-gangliosidosis[71]

Clinical aspects

This disorder of autosomal recessive inheritance usually presents as Tay–Sachs disease at around 6 months of age, but is occasionally observed in young adults. The presentation is predominantly neurological, although sometimes behavioural change, intellectual decline and a slowly developing dementia are found. There are several other types of G_{M2}-gangliosidosis apart from this one, namely Tay–Sachs disease, Sandhoff's disease, and juvenile G_{M2}-gangliosidosis.

Biochemical basis

There is accumulation of G_{M2}-ganglioside in the engorged lysosomes of the neurones in both the central and autonomic nervous system, due to deficiency of hexosaminidase A, which catalyses conversion of G_{M2}-ganglioside to G_{M3}-ganglioside

Neuronal ceroid lipofuscinosis[71]

Clinical aspects

This lipid storage disease of autosomal recessive inheritance presents in adolescence or early adult life (the latter form is also referred to as Kufs disease). The other neurolipidoses are sphingomyelin lipidosis (Niemann–Pick disease), glucosyl ceramide lipidosis (Gaucher's disease), and the various gangliosidoses. In addition to neurological features there is, initially, intellectual deterioration with learning difficulties and progression to dementia.

Biochemical basis

Neuropathologically, there is cerebral atrophy with lipopigment accumulation in the form of ceroid or lipofuscin within the lysosomes and in other parts of the body. The biochemical basis of the condition is uncertain. However, neuronal accumulation of lipofuscin does occur normally with increasing age – and it could be that lipofuscin deposition is one of the causes of memory loss at this time of life.

Subacute necrotizing encephalopathy (Leigh's disease)

Clinical aspects[71]

This disorder of autosomal recessive inheritance may, very rarely, begin as late as adolescence and consists of neurological features accompanied by psychomotor retardation and impaired intellectual function, usually of mild degree.

Biochemical basis[71]

Biochemically there is gross depletion of serum pyruvate carboxylase, the enzyme which normally converts pyruvate to oxaloacetate; as a result there are increased concentrations of pyruvate, lactate and alanine in body fluids, together with a metabolic acidosis. Neuropathologically there is widespread cellular necrosis in the brain with capillary proliferation; the distribution of lesions is similar to that of Wernicke's encephalopathy.

7
Psychiatric side-effects of drugs, plants, fungi and dinoflagellates

PSYCHIATRIC SIDE-EFFECTS OF DRUG THERAPY

Psychiatric changes attributable solely (or in part) to commencement, continuation or cessation of drug therapy range from mere changes of mood to much more florid clinical presentations. The interactions of a drug, not only with the personality but also with physiological status and metabolic inheritance (i.e. pharmacogenetic aspects) of the individual, are fundamental to the actual clinical expression of toxicity; the dosage, too, is a vital consideration. The elderly often have cerebral atherosclerosis and may be more sensitive to the effects of drugs; moreover, concomitant presence of alcohol may produce an additive effect – or just complicate the presentation. With a psychiatric illness in particular it is often very difficult to be certain that the patient's symptoms are related to the drug therapy – as opposed to being due to an exacerbation or phase of the original clinical problem. This applies whether it is the presence of the drug or its withdrawal that is being incriminated.

The psychiatric manifestations of adverse responses to drugs include schizophrenic-like reactions (paranoia), depression, hypomania, hallucinations, delirium (confusion), sleep disturbance and drowsiness; symptoms of lesser severity are, however, very common and singly (or collectively) may be significantly incapacitating. In addition to these definitive reactions there are those even less well defined complaints where the patient claims that 'the tablets made me feel awful'; in these cases it may well be that the individual lacks the ability and clarity of thought to be able to precisely define and clearly articulate his feelings.

It is not the intention here to provide a comprehensive list of adverse psychiatric accompaniments of drug therapy; nevertheless, some of the more common symptoms are quoted, together with a few of the more unusual ones – merely to provide a more complete spectrum of the feelings that are, from time to time, reported.

NON-PSYCHOTROPIC DRUGS

Benzhexol (an antimuscarinic drug used in parkinsonism) can cause nervousness, confusion, excitement and severe psychiatric disturbance.

Chlorpropamide (a sulphonylurea compound) both stimulates and potentiates the action of antidiuretic hormone (ADH), causing SIADH (and all its associated mood changes) in rare instances; many other drugs, likewise, can cause this syndrome (Chapter 6).

Cytosine arabinoside (an antimetabolite used in the therapy of certain leukaemias) in high dosage may produce personality changes, somnolence, coma, vivid and peculiar nightmares; some patients complain of having 'odd thoughts'.

Digoxin (a cardiac glycoside, possessing positive inotropic actions) sometimes causes confusion, disorientation and hallucinations; other more occasional observations are of agitation, excitement, disturbance of sleep, weakness, apathy and depression.

α-Interferon (a naturally occurring protein with antiviral ant-proliferative and immuno-modulatory activity) can make the patient very depressed, perhaps accompanied by suicidal thoughts; milder symptoms include lassitude, tiredness and general malaise.

Levodopa (a dopaminergic compound) can generate mild elation, depression, anxiety, agitation, aggression, hallucinations and delusions.

Methyldopa (a centrally acting antihypertensive drug) may produce tiredness and exhaustion.

Prazocin (an α-adrenoreceptor blocking agent) sometimes causes drowsiness, lack of energy, weakness and anxiety.

Prednisone (and other adrenal corticosteroid analogues) can cause mild euphoria, hyperactivity, sleeplessness, disorientation, confusion and sometimes a frank psychosis (e.g. hypomania).

Propanolol (and other β-adrenoreceptor blocking agents) commonly produce mental lassitude, loss of motivation, lack of mental agility (e.g. inability to maintain a conversation on account of failure to recall full details of the discussion as it proceeds), impairment of short-term recall (whereas long-term memory is unaffected), exhaustion and lack of energy. Sudden withdrawal of the drug can lead to anxiety of severe degree.

Salbutamol (a selective β$_2$-adrenoreceptor stimulant), when given to asthmatic patients, can provoke a reaction which at first appears to be anxiety; on analysis, however, it is a tenseness and tremor of skeletal muscle origin and not due to direct CNS stimulation.

Theophylline (a potent CNS stimulant) can, in excess, stimulate odd dreams and sleep disturbance.

Thyroxine (one of the thyroid hormones) in high doses, can lead to anxiety and insomnia.

CASE 15[94]

Clinical history

A ten-and-a-half year old boy was admitted to hospital as an emergency with a 3 h history of confusion, hyperactivity, restlessness, visual hallucinations and short-term memory loss; he was apyrexial. He had been at home with his father over the preceding 5 h. He had no known allergies, was not on any medication and, on direct questioning, denied taking any drugs. His mother was receiving fluoxetine, dothiepin and lithium carbonate treatment for her longstanding depression but insisted that none of her tablets were missing. It was revealed that one year earlier the boy had deliberately ingested his mother's antibiotics, but his parents were convinced that he would not have repeated such an episode. Later, it was confirmed that he was on the Child Protection Register on account of previous physical abuse by his father.

Clinical examination revealed an apyrexial, confused and restless child with obvious pressure of speech and confabulation – interspersed with some normal speech; his buccal mucosa was dry. The pulse rate was regular at 120 beats per minute and the blood pressure was 114/60 mmHg. His pupils were dilated and reacted sluggishly to light;

---

there was absence of meningism and no cranial nerve palsies were detected.

Laboratory investigations

Serum urea, electrolytes, liver function tests and thyroid function tests were all within the reference ranges; the full blood count, urinalysis and electroencephalogram (EEG) were all within normal limits. An electrocardiogram showed sinus tachycardia without any evidence of arrhythmia; both blood and urine cultures were subsequently revealed to be sterile.

Analysis and comments

A provisional diagnosis of psychosis secondary to drug ingestion, with a differential diagnosis of viral encephalitis, was made following consultation with a Child Psychiatrist. Atropine-like signs and symptoms suggested the possibility of hyoscine poisoning and direct questioning revealed that travel sickness tablets had been purchased by the family 2 years earlier. His mother was persuaded to return to the house to check the cupboard for medications; the search revealed an empty blister pack which originally held 10 tablets, each containing 300 µg of hyoscine hydrobromide. She was adamant that only 2 tablets had ever been used, so 8 tablets were now missing. Analysis of the urine sample taken on admission confirmed the presence of hyoscine and its degradation products. The patient, however, continued to deny ingesting any tablets at all and, more specifically, the hyoscine-containing travel sickness tablets; he was discharged 2 days later after making a full recovery.

A diagnosis of viral encephalitis had initially been considered possible, although unlikely because the child remained apyrexial without further progression of symptoms and with a normal EEG. The features were thought to be more compatible with overdose of an atropine-like drug which could cause drying of secretions, tachycardia, hypertension and dilated pupils, together with hallucinations, behavioural abnormalities and short-term memory loss (central anticholinergic syndrome). Although fluoxetine can cause similar symptoms it results in hypotension, fever and excessive sweating and was, therefore, considered unlikely to be the responsible agent. Dothiepin possesses anti-muscarinic effects but is less likely to cause the central anticholinergic syndrome. Many of the features of lithium carbonate toxicity were absent and there was no convincing evidence to implicate this compound. Some travel sickness tablets contain hyoscine hydrobromide and are commonly found at home as they are so easily available over-the-counter. On account of both clinical suspicion and circumstantial evidence pointing towards possible ingestion of travel sickness tablets the request for toxicological studies on the urine for hyoscine specifically, rather than a general toxicology screen, saved both time and money.

The reasons for deliberate drug ingestion in this case remain unclear. Lack of parental supervision may have been a contributory factor to his excursion into experimenting with drugs. His continued denial, despite evidence to the contrary, may have been part of the amnesia associated with hyoscine or it could have been deliberate because he might have feared an angry reaction from his father following discharge; another possibility was that he felt obliged to perpetuate the lie he had, perhaps, formulated initially. Munchausen-by-proxy was also considered. Social Services were informed of the episode and the Child Psychiatrist offered follow-up in order to explore and discuss any possible family problems.

Hyoscine is a potentially fatal drug that is easily available over-the-counter and may, in consequence, be perceived by lay persons as being minimally harmful. Drug ingestion should, therefore, be considered a possibility in all cases presenting with toxic confusional state even in the face of denial by the patient and disbelief by the parents. The psychological/psychiatric component of a clinical history should always be appraised carefully as therein may lie a vital clue to the proper diagnosis. It should be emphasized that hyoscine toxicity, either deliberate or accidental, is a well recognized entity not only in adults but also in children. Acute life-threatening episodes (ALTE) have been reported to result from both transdermal patches and colic medications. Every travel sickness medication containing hyoscine hydrobromide should, surely, carry a cautionary label on each pack. Furthermore, a clear clinical history is vitally important – not only in aiding the differentiation of acute viral infections involving the central nervous system (such as acute encephalitis) from drug toxicity, but also in rationalizing any further diagnostic investigations.

PSYCHOTROPIC DRUGS[95,96]

Anxiolytic drugs

Clinical aspects

Benzodiazepines (e.g. diazepam, lorazepam, oxazepam, chlordiaze-poxide, lormetazepam, flurazepam, temazepam, clonazepam, etc.) as a group can cause drowsiness, sedation, unsteadiness, ataxia, confusion and occasional aggressive outbursts with excitement. Excessive or prolonged use of these compounds may lead to psychological dependency, with the consequence of withdrawal symptoms following abrupt discontinuation of therapy. This may produce increased anxiety, tension, headache, confusion, insomnia and perceptual disturbances – with, in severe cases, depression and paranoid ideation.

Non-benzodiazepine anxiolytic compounds include **buspirone, chlormezanone, hydroxyzine, meprobamate** and others. **Buspirone** can cause mild symptoms at the beginning of therapy, subsiding later; they include nervousness, excitement, drowsiness, fatigue, light-headedness, headache and confusion. **Chlormezanone** may produce drowsiness and lethargy. **Hydroxyzine** only occasionally produces mental side-effects, comprising slightly impaired ability in performing tasks, weakness, confusion and transitory drowsiness in the first few days. **Meprobamate** commonly produces drowsiness and sedation; alertness may be impaired, whereas excitement and euphoria are reported from time to time.

Mechanisms of action

Benzodiazepines act on the CNS mainly through inhibiting the $GABA_A$ neurotransmitter receptors, normally activated by GABA. *Non-benzodiazepine* compounds act in different ways. **Buspirone,** one of the azapirones (azaspirodecanediones), is a non-benzodiazepine anxiolytic compound which binds with inhibitory $5HT_{1A}$-autoreceptors on 5HT cell bodies, thus decreasing 5HT neurotransmission. **Chlormezanone** is reserved for short-term use in anxiety. **Hydroxyzine** is an antihistamine compound, only effective for anxiety in sedative doses. **Meprobamate** is one of the propanediol carbamates. β-Adrenergic receptor antagonists, such as **propanolol,** are not effective in the management of generalized anxiety or panic states – but they are able to lessen autonomic symptoms that may occur in specific situational phobias.

Antidepressant drugs

Clinical aspects

Tricyclic compounds (e.g. **amitriptyline, mianserin,** etc.) are listed as sometimes causing different degrees of confusion, disturbed concentration, drowsiness, cognitive impairment, disorientation, delusions, hallucinations, hypomania, excitement, anxiety, restlessness, insomnia and nightmares.

Modified tricyclic compounds (e.g. **lofepramine, amoxapine,** etc.) sometimes produce anxiety and insomnia.

Sedative tricyclic compounds (e.g. **mianserin, trazodone**) may cause sedation and cognitive impairment.

Monoamine oxidase inhibitor (MAOI) drugs (e.g. **phenelzine, isocarboxazid, tranylcypromine, moclobemide** etc.) can produce drowsiness, weakness, fatigue, insomnia, nervousness, euphoria and behavioural changes; MAOI drugs interact with foods containing tyramine – and with other drugs (e.g. sympathomimetics, selective serotonin re-uptake inhibitors and opiates). **Moclobemide** has no risk of the dietary reaction associated with tyramine-containing foods, but may still be associated with potentiation of sympathetic compounds and opiates.

Selective serotonin re-uptake inhibitor (SSRI) drugs (e.g. **fluvoxamine, fluoxetine, paroxetine, sertraline,** etc.) may lead to drowsiness, dizziness, headache, agitation, anxiety, fatigue and insomnia.

Serotonin noradrenaline re-uptake inhibitor (SNRI) drugs (e.g. **venlafaxine**) can cause insomnia, somnolence, dizziness, nervousness and anxiety.

Miscellaneous drugs include **tryptophan,** unrelated to the tricyclic or MAOI compounds; this can cause drowsiness. **Nefazodone** and **trazodone** are atypical antidepressants; nefazodone resembles trazodone pharmacologically but is less sedating.

Mechanisms of action

Most of the **tricyclic antidepressant** (TCA) compounds, i.e. tertiary amine tricyclics (e.g. **amitriptylene, clomipramine, doxepin, imipramine**) and secondary amine tricyclics (e.g. **desipramine, maprotiline, nortriptylene**) potently antagonize acetylcholine receptors, H_1-histamine receptors and α_1-adrenoceptors; they also, in varying degrees, inhibit both 5HT and NA re-uptake. **Clomipramine** is a TCA compound which potently inhibits 5HT re-uptake; it does, therefore, potently potentiate 5HT – and NA transmission, as also does **venlafaxine**. **Trazodone** and **mianserin** block H_1-histamine receptors and α_1-adrenoceptors – but not acetylcholine receptors. **Monoamine oxidase inhibitor** (MAOI) drugs inhibit monoamine oxidase (MAO) types A and B; **moclobemide**, however, reversibly inhibits MAO type A. **Selective serotonin re-uptake inhibitor** (SSRI) compounds block 5HT re-uptake. **Serotonin noradrenaline re-uptake inhibitor** (SNRI) drugs, e.g. **venlafaxine**, directly inhibits both 5HT (SSRI action) and NA re-uptake. **Nefazodone** one of the miscellaneous drugs does not antagonize α_1-adrenoceptors; it weakly inhibits 5HT re-uptake, but selectively blocks $5HT_2$ receptors – it probably facilitates $5HT_{1A}$ neurotransmission via both these mechanisms.

Antipsychotic drugs

Clinical aspects

Phenothiazines comprise three groups of drugs – the aliphatic compounds of group 1 (e.g. **chlorpromazine, promazine**, etc.), the piperidine compounds of group 2 (e.g. **pericyazine, thioridazine**, etc.) and the piperazine compounds of group 3 (e.g. **fluphenazine, trifluoperazine**, etc.). The sedative effects, being maximum in group 1, decline through groups 2 and 3.

Other antipsychotic compounds tend to resemble the group 3 phenothiazines. They include butyrophenones (e.g. **droperidol, haloperidol**, etc.), diphenylbutylpiperidines (e.g. **fluspirilene, pimozide**, etc.), thioxanthenes (e.g. **flupenthixol, zuclopenthixol**, etc.) and oxypertine, whereas the benzamide compounds (e.g. **sulpiride, remoxipride**, etc.) are structurally distinct from the other antipsychotic drugs. In general, the sedative effects of all the latter tend to be less than for the group 1 phenothiazines; however, agitation and hyperactivity can occur with oxypertine in low doses. **Risperidone** a benzisoxazole derivative, is a heterocyclic neuroleptic; it can cause insomnia, anxiety, headache, somnolence, fatigue, dizziness and difficulty in concentration.

Mechanisms of action

The mechanism of action of antipsychotic drugs is by way of their effective blockade of dopamine D_2-receptors in the mesolimbic and mesocortical areas of the brain; **clozapine**, however, is not an effective dopamine D_2-receptor blocker. D_2-receptor blockade in the basal ganglia is the cause of extrapyramidal movement disorders sometimes seen as an adverse effect of such therapy. **Haloperidol** and **fluphenazine** are selective antagonists of dopamine receptors, but **chlorpromazine** and **thioridazine** possess, in addition to their dopamine receptor blocking properties, the ability to block acetylcholine receptors, H_1-histamine receptors and α_1-adrenoceptors. **Sulpiride** is a highly selective D_2-receptor antagonist. **Risperidone** potently antagonizes $5HT_2$-receptors as well as D_2-receptors.

Mood stabilizing drugs

Clinical aspects

Lithium carbonate toxicity progresses through apathy, mild drowsiness, clouding of consciousness, impairment of memory and agitation; coma occurs in severe overdosage, whereas sudden cessation of therapy can precipitate hypomania or mania.

Carbamazepine can produce side-effects of headache, drowsiness and dizziness.

Sodium valproate can produce the toxic effect of drowsiness.

Mechanisms of action

Lithium is a small ion that affects the functions of amines such as NA, DA, 5HT; it also affects sodium and potassium flux across cell membranes, causes a decrease in the liberation of inositol from inositol phosphate by inhibiting the phosphatase enzyme that governs this reaction and may modify the amount and function of G proteins and effectors. **Carbamazepine** and **valproic acid** have similar actions to phenytoin, in that they all inhibit repetitive firing of cortical and spinal neurones – probably by decreasing the recovery rate of voltage-activated sodium channels from a state of inactivation.

DRUGS OF ABUSE AND THEIR PSYCHIATRIC EFFECTS[74,97]

These compounds will be discussed under the headings of opioid analgesics, CNS depressants, CNS stimulants, cannabis, psychedelic drugs and inhalants.

Opioid (narcotic) analgesics[97]

Heroin (diamorphine, diacetyl morphine), more potent than morphine, also causes euphoria and addiction.

Methadone is less sedating than morphine.

Morphine administration causes euphoria, dependence and tolerance.

Pentazocine is able to induce hallucinations and thought disturbance.

Opiate compounds exert their effects by binding with opiate receptors, which are particularly well represented in the limbic system. It was the discovery of these receptors that led in the first place to the discovery of the endogenous morphine-like peptides in the CNS, the gastrointestinal tract (enkephalins) and the pituitary gland (endorphins). These endogenous morphine-like compounds produce analgesia, tolerance and dependence. Enkephalins are involved in the pathways of pain, affective states and appetite control. Anxiety and panic, a feature of opiate withdrawal, may be caused by overactivity of the noradrenergic system.

CNS depressants[97]

Alcohol (p. 142) and **benzodiazepines** (p. 147) have been discussed already.

Amitriptyline has also been discussed (p. 148).

Bromides are still sometimes found in proprietary preparations and can accumulate over a period of many weeks to give bromism. Symptoms include irritability, drowsiness, lethargy, impaired memory, interference with thought processes and ultimately confusion, hallucinations and coma.

Methyprylone, a piperidinedione derivative, can cause paradoxical excitement and confusion prior to sleep.

CNS stimulants[97]

Amphetamines, which are more powerful CNS stimulants than caffeine, induce feelings of alertness, well-being, euphoria and exhilaration, together with anxiety, tension and tremor as the dose increases. In some cases of amphetamine abuse, amphetamine psychosis occurs; it is almost indistinguishable from acute schizophrenic illness.

Caffeine (a methylxanthine compound) can, in small doses, promote more rapid (and clearer) flow of thought, but over-indulgence can lead to nervousness, restlessness and insomnia; it is a weak CNS stimulant.

Cocaine has psychoactive effects, comprising feelings of immense energy, alertness and confidence, with increased activity and incessant talking, in addition to irritability, anxiety and suspiciousness. The euphoria is of short-term duration on account of acute and chronic tolerance. Cessation of the drug can lead to apathy, fatigue, depression and sleep. Cocaine interferes with reuptake of catecholamines at adrenergic nerve endings, thus potentiating sympathetic nervous system activity. Metabolism of cocaine proceeds via plasma esterases, the metabolites being excreted in the urine.

Diethylpropion can cause insomnia, nervousness, psychosis, hallucinations and dependence.

Cannabis (marijuana, hashish)[97]

Δ-9-tetrahydrocannabinol (THC) is the main psychoactive component of cannabis. It can induce mild euphoria, some depression of consciousness, distortion of the sense of time, fragmentation of thought processes and hallucinations. Higher doses lead to perplexity, ecstasy, feelings of depersonalization and derealization, episodes of panic and even frank terror.

Psychedelic drugs[97]

These compounds, variously called hallucinogens, psychotogens and psychotomimetics, produce distortion of perception, thought, feeling and behaviour. Under this group of compounds comes **lysergic acid diethylamide (LSD)**, **psilocybin** ('magic mushrooms'), **psilocin**, **dimethyltryptamine (DMT)**, **diethyltryptamine (DET)**, **mescaline**, **2,5-dimethoxy-4-methyl-amphetamine (DOM)**, the anticholinergic compounds (i.e. the alkaloids **atropine**, **hyoscyamine** and **scopolamine**), **phencyclidine** ('angel dust', **PCP**) and **ketamine**. The psychiatric effects induced by all these compounds are very similar to those produced by LSD. 5HT (particularly $5HT_2$) receptors are the sites at which hallucinogenic drugs act.

Lysergic acid diethylamide (LSD) is a psychedelic drug which produces distortion of perception (e.g. body image), thought, feeling and behaviour, together with vivid hallucinations (particularly visual ones), lability of mood, states of panic and sudden outbursts of anger. The individual may, for instance, think he/she is a bird and jump from a great height with outstretched arms. Chronic usage of the compound may induce derangements of memory and can create difficulties with problem solving and abstract thought. Schizophrenic-like psychoses may be precipitated, and there can be 'flash-backs' occasionally, up to many months following exposure. At low dosage, there is vasospasm of the cerebral arteries. LSD acts mainly at $5HT_2$ receptor sites.

Phencyclidine ('angel dust', PCP), a hallucinogen, is a cyclohexylamine derivative. The psychiatric consequences include agitation, excitement, distortion of body image perception, disorganization of thought and feelings of estrangement. The presentation can mimic an acute schizophrenic reaction. There is a high risk of suicide and of aggression with violence. Chronic administration causes insomnia, behavioural changes, social problems and chronic schizophrenia. At low doses the drug produces vasospasm of the cerebral arteries.

153

Inhalants[97]

Inhalants comprise organic solvents (e.g. **toluene**), **amyl nitrite**, **nitrous oxide** and many other compounds. In general, they produce a rapid onset of dizziness, intoxication, activity, euphoria, hilarity and sometimes loss of consciousness.

PSYCHIATRIC EFFECTS OF PLANTS, FUNGI AND DINOFLAGELLATES

Many of the compounds referred to in the sections entitled 'Psychiatric side-effects of drug therapy' (p. 142) and 'Drugs of abuse and their psychiatric effects' (p. 151) are identical (or, chemically, closely related) to substances of botanical origin. In this section discussion will centre around the effects of directly ingesting the poisonous plants (or parts thereof) themselves. Neurotoxin-producing dinoflagellates (which, in turn, contaminate shellfish) and poisonous fungi will also be included. There must, necessarily, be some crossover with pharmacognosy, the subject that is largely concerned with the study of naturally occurring substances with medicinal properties (or, alternatively, which serve as safe flavouring agents, suspending agents, etc.); many of these are of botanical origin, but some are from sources within the animal kingdom. Some plant compounds, being toxic only in high doses, might be medicinal at low dosage; yet others are toxic even in small amounts. The examples which follow have been selected for their general interest and range, bearing in mind that a comprehensive list would be outside the scope of this review. Moreover, symptoms other than changes of mood have been specifically omitted from these entries.

Poisonous plants[98]

Black nightshade (*Solanum nigrum*) can cause trembling and coma if the attractive looking berries are eaten. Solanine is the alkaloid present, the amount varying with the nature of the soil, the season and the geographical location.

Deadly nightshade (*Atropa belladonna*) can cause excitement, drowsiness, hallucinations and coma if the berries are ingested. The alkaloids hyoscyamine, atropine and hyoscine are the toxic agents.

154

Hemlock (*Conium maculatum*) poisoning can cause mental confusion, coma and death. The alkaloids coniine, cohydrine, N-methyconiine and coniceine are present in all parts of the plant and may be largely responsible for the symptoms.

Laburnum (*Laburnum anagyroides*) can, in sufficient dosage, cause restlessness, drowsiness and delirium. The toxic alkaloid cytisine is present in all parts of the tree.

Monkshood (*Aconitum napellus*) ingestion can cause restlessness, convulsions and death. Aconitine, a narcotic alkaloid, is the chief toxic agent of the plant which is present in roots and leaves.

Nutmeg, the dried kernels of the seeds of *Myristica fragrans* (Myristicaceae), from which the volatile oil 'nutmeg oil' is obtained by distillation, in large doses causes euphoria, drowsiness, disorientation, depersonalization, feelings of remoteness and hallucinations; these symptoms are thought to be due to the hallucinogens myristicin and elemicin.

The **opium poppy** (*Papaver somniferum*) is grown in many countries for the purpose of extracting opium which produces narcotic effects. Opium contains in excess of 25 alkaloids (chief amongst which are morphine, codeine, thebaine, noscopine, narceine and papaverine), together with sugars, sulphates, colouring matter, albuminous substances, etc.

Potato (*Solanum tuberosum*), if green, can cause confusion, hallucinations and coma following eating. The alkaloidal glycosides (α-solanine and α-chaconine) responsible for the symptoms, and normally present only in small amounts in the peel, increase in amount during the greening and sprouting which follows either exposure of the potato tubers to light or storage under adverse conditions.

The **Peyotl** (*Lophophora williamsii*), a cactus long used by the Mexican Indians in their religious ceremonies, produces hallucinations following ingestion. The chief constituent responsible is the alkaloid mescaline.

Thornapple (*Datura stramonium*) poisoning leads to delirium, coma and death. The alkaloids atropine, hyoscine and hyoscyamine are present in all parts of the plant, particularly the seeds.

Yew (*Taxus baccata*) produces delirium and coma following ingestion of the leaves and seeds; an alkaloid is responsible.

CASE 16[99]

Clinical history

A 20-year-old male, previously in good health, had been in the company of five other males and one female drinking alcohol one afternoon in a small country town in Australia. They then all left by car and travelled into the bush, having picked up flowers from a deserted garden on the way. At their destination they divided the flowers and proceeded to eat them. There is uncertainty regarding exactly what happened after that, except that the 20-year-old was found dead 40 h later, lying face upwards in water just 1 foot deep.

Laboratory investigations

Urine tests for atropine, scopolamine and hyoscyamine were not performed in this case, but there is indication that the tests would have been positive, as in the stomach at postmortem examination were found remnants of the flowers and stems that he had eaten. They were later identified as being from *Datura arborea* ('The Angel's Trumpet', 'Trumpet Lilies'). No other drugs were identified in the blood, urine or body fluids. Death was thought to have occurred < 24 h previously, probably on the same night that the flower eating session had taken place.

Analysis and comments

All except two individuals returned to their homes 24 h later. The full story emerged from one of them; he was dazed, in great agitation, disorientated, perspiring, and was terrified. He was noted to have dilated pupils. As he recovered he was able to describe the whole fearful experience, providing a vivid account of how he imagined trees and people chasing him with weapons, including guns and spears.

From his account the police identified the site and found one of the two lost males standing by a eucalyptus tree, talking to it lovingly, although when disturbed he stared at them unrespondingly. He thought that one of the group was lying on the ground nearby, but when the police investigated they found what was merely a discarded coat.

It is known that intoxication with *Datura* plants can produce a variety of symptoms and signs including dryness of the mouth, thirst, feeling hot, dilatation of the pupils, visual problems, frightening hallucinations, flushing, palpitations, tachycardia, ataxia, delirium and coma – with cardiac and respiratory arrest as the terminal event.

In the case of the dead male, theories put forward to explain the series of events were either: (i) that the 'thirst and heat' feeling caused him to enter the water to cool off and obtain a drink, at which point he had a cardiac arrest, or (ii) that he had deliberately submerged himself in the water, with intent to seek refuge from his imaginary pursuers. The literature refers to other similar cases where individuals have been found swimming – looking for red-eyed dolphins! There is also the possibility that there might have been some exacerbation of effect of the toxins in the presence of alcohol.

The genus *Datura* belongs to the *Solanum* family, which includes many plants with hypnotic properties, e.g. mandrake (*Mandragora officinarum*), deadly nightshade (*Atropa belladonna*) and henbane (*Hyoscyamus niger*). From these plants have been isolated various tropane alkaloids, including scopolamine, hyoscyamine, norhyoscyamine, meteloidine and atropine, all of which vary in amount and proportion, depending not only on the actual part of the plant being analysed but also on the stage of maturation.

Poisonous fungi[98]

Some fungi contain psychoactive compounds; they include bufotoxin, psilocin and mescaline.

Fly Agaric (*Amanita muscaria*) is a mushroom which, following ingestion, produces hallucinations; it contains hallucinogenic substances.

Liberty Cap (*Psilocybe semilanceate*), together with *Panaeolus foenisecii*, can cause hallucinations; both these mushrooms contain the hallucinogen psilocybin, each of them having been taken at various times with the specific intention of producing these effects.

Dinoflagellates[100]

Shellfish poisoning, e.g. from bivalve molluscs contaminated with neurotoxins synthesized by dinoflagellates (such as *Gonyaulax catanella* and *Gonyaulax tamarensis*), can produce (amongst other symptoms) a 'feeling of floating'. Saxitoxin is the neurotoxin produced by *Gonyaulax catanella*.

8
Munchausen syndrome and related disorders

The disorders discussed hitherto have all been psychiatric, secondary to biochemical, pharmacological and clinical events[101]. In this section discussion will centre on those conditions in which the psychological state, together with its surrounding circumstances, precede the 'biochemistry'. An example would be the patient who takes non-prescribed medication (or one which has been prescribed, but taken in deliberately wrong dosage) with the knowledge that symptoms and/or signs will result, which will in turn secondarily serve as a diagnostic challenge to the doctors with the possible ultimate spin-off that care, attention and interest will be shown. Other instances where metallic and other objects have been ingested are variants of the same theme, but such presentations are somewhat peripheral to the scope of this discussion.

MALINGERING, FACTITIOUS DISORDERS AND DISSOCIATIVE DISORDERS (HYSTERIA)[102,103]

Before proceeding it should be recognized that there is a spectrum of disorders ranging from malingering at one end, through factitious disorders (including Munchausen syndrome) to (hysteria) at the other. Moreover, it is necessary at this point to provide a brief definition of each of these conditions, in order that Munchausen syndrome may be seen in proper perspective.

Malingering involves the faking of an illness with intent to obtain some tangible reward (e.g. pethidine injections, monetary compensation, time off work or avoidance of a potentially unenviable circumstance). These people, often prisoners or military personnel, who fraudulently claim symptoms or exaggerate their already present clinical disorder, are fully aware of their motivation and know that they are intentionally faking the situation.

Factitious disorders comprise deliberate production of physical and/or psychological symptoms, but without either an obvious external incentive or identifiable reward; there just seems to be a psychological requirement to perpetuate the scenario of 'sickness'.

Munchausen syndrome is an extreme form of the disorder, with the seeking of attention for some reason (e.g. the patient may need love, care, attention, or sympathy), hence choosing to 'create illness' in order to achieve this end. Such individuals are not aware of their motivation, but fully realize that they are faking a clinical presentation. In the '**Munchausen syndrome by proxy**', it is usually the parents (often the mother) who seek medical help, falsely representing the child's symptoms, sometimes even making false physical signs and interfering, too, with biological specimens to be sent for laboratory analysis (e.g. they might add glucose to the urine sample, etc.).

Dissociative disorders (hysteria) is where the patient is consciously unaware that the illness is simulated; moreover, there seems to be no obvious gain – indeed, there could even be financial loss, discomfort or pain as a consequence. The patient is not aware of motivation or of intentionally faking the situation. There may be dissociative and conversion symptoms; dissociative symptoms comprise amnesia, multiple personality and fugue states, whereas conversion symptoms may include anaesthesia, aphonia, convulsions and blindness.

THE PATIENT WITH MUNCHAUSEN SYNDROME

Patients with Munchausen syndrome may, from time to time, present to clinicians in any discipline of medicine. These people are typically lonely, having few or no visitors, often reported by the ward nursing staff as 'being strange' or 'behaving oddly' and with apparent inappropriately less concern for their 'illness' than might be expected, had it been genuine. Nevertheless, they often enquire regularly as to the progress being made in sorting out their diagnosis. The clinical features are often bizarre, perhaps causing much curiosity and interest before the suspicion arises that the disorder is not of natural origin. It is important to establish the patient's background, interests (particularly regarding biology) and education; many do have some medical knowledge. On examination there may be scars of previous abdominal operations which they may attribute to severe injury at some time in the past. Their stay in hospital may be short and they frequently discharge themselves against medical advice, and sometimes without any warning at all.

It is always time well spent to check the basic data these people have provided (e.g. their home address, the name and address of their general practitioner, etc.); very often such information is erroneous – and may, in fact, be far from the location at which they present. Sometimes, however, no such information is forthcoming as it has been 'forgotten'. For a patient to forget such basic facts might be judged as being out of expectation for the individual, particularly when viewed in the context of all the supposedly accurate information that has already been confidently provided. Important clues and information may, if they are sought, also come from casual remarks dropped by the patient to those who tend them (e.g. nurses, venepuncturists, physiotherapists, etc.), which although on their own are seemingly trivial and of no significance, yet collectively could provide very valuable corroborative data.

CASE 17

Clinical history

A 36-year-old lady was admitted to hospital on 30.03.73 with a 3-month history of colicky abdominal pain radiating to the right hypochondrium, together with vomiting. The pain usually started 10 min after taking food or fluid, lasted for about half an hour and was relieved by vomiting. She said that she had had an attack of jaundice a few months earlier. Her past history included a hysterectomy for menorrhagia in 1962 and an emergency operation in 1967 during which her 'stomach was stitched'. In 1971 she was diagnosed as having a bleeding peptic ulcer for which an emergency abdominal operation was performed, although according to the records no evidence of peptic ulceration or biliary disease had been found.

On examination she was grossly obese, was not in great pain and was not jaundiced; she was, however, tender over the right side of the abdomen. There was no pyrexia. The possibility of cholecystitis was considered, although subsequent extensive investigations were all negative.

Near to the point of discharge, however, she was found to have a positive Benedict's test on routine urine analysis. On direct questioning she admitted to having had diabetes mellitus previously, but said that it had 'now got better'. There had been no evidence of this at the time of admission to the surgical ward.

Laboratory investigations

Date	Time (24 h)	Plasma 'glucose' (mmol/l)	Serum osmolality (mosmol/kg)	Urine osmolality (mosmol/kg)	Urine testing B	C	K
13.04.73	–	8.2	–	–	+	–	+
16.04.73	–	2.5	–	–			
17.04.73	10.00	49.7	–	–			
		5.2*	290	–			
	12.15	3.4*	287	–			
	14.50	4.8*	288	–			
02.05.73	11.00	26.1	–	805			
		3.9*					
09.05.73	09.00	4.7	–	1148	+	+	–
		5.0*					

N.B. * = Glucose oxidase method (all other tests were done by a method which measured reducing substances). B = Benedict's test, C = Clinistix, K = ketones

Date	Glucose load (g)	Plasma 'glucose' values (mmol/l) 0 h	0.5 h	1.0 h	1.5 h	2.0 h	Urine testing B	C	K
13.04.73	50	6.3	23.0	78.9	66.7	27.3	+	–	+
14.04.73	50	33.7	19.0	36.4	57.8	40.0	+	–	+
26.04.73	2	32.3	33.8	65.8	25.0	40.8	+	–	+
02.05.73	5	31.7	32.2	26.2	33.3	26.1			
		6.0*	5.9*	5.6*	4.4*	3.9*			
09.05.73	10	4.7	–	32.2	50.0	66.7	+	+	–
		5.0*	31.7*	46.7*	46.7	60.1	+	+	–

N.B. * = Glucose oxidase method (all other tests were done by a method which measured reducing substances). B = Benedict's test, C = Clinistix, K = ketones

162

Initially, on 02.04.73, the serum sodium concentration was 140 mmol/l (RR 135–147), the serum potassium was 3.9 mmol/l (RR 3.5–5.0), serum chloride 96 mmol/l (RR 95–107), serum bicarbonate 28 mmol/l (RR 21–30) and serum urea 1.0 mmol/l (RR 2.5–6.5). The serum bilirubin was 5 μmol/l (RR 2–17), total protein 61 g/l (RR 60–80), serum albumin 37 g/l (RR 35–40), serum AP 48 IU/l (RR 30–125) and serum AST 43 IU/l (RR 7–40); the protein electrophoresis was within normal limits. A cholecystogram was reported as 'the gall bladder concentrated the dye well and has contracted satisfactorily after a fatty meal. No stones are noted'. An intravenous pyelogram was reported as normal.

Comments and analysis

The urine samples continued to be positive for reducing substances, but the plasma 'glucose' done by a method which measured reducing substances was 8.2 mmol/l. Nevertheless, a glucose tolerance test (GTT) following administration of 50 g glucose was performed on 13.04.73. It revealed a bizarre pattern of plasma 'glucose' levels starting at 6.3 mmol/l, rising to 23.0 mmol/l at 0.5 h and reaching 78.9 mmol/l at 1.0 h, subsequently falling to 66.7 mmol/l at 1.5 h and 27.3 mmol/l at 2.0 h. The urine samples throughout the test were positive for both reducing substances and ketones, but negative when tested with Clinistix. A repeat test the next day was similar, but did not show the rise and fall as clearly. On 17.04.73 the true plasma glucose value, measured using the glucose oxidase method, revealed a value of 5.2 mmol/l at a time when the plasma 'glucose' was 49.7 mmol/l, although serum osmolality values were within the reference range; hence, the reducing substance was, clearly, not glucose. Chromatography of the urine on 17.04.73 revealed the presence of large amounts of lactose. On 02.05.73 a further GTT, using a loading dose of 5 g glucose, was performed; this revealed a very similar pattern to the previous tests. However, when the same samples were subjected to the glucose oxidase method there was a flat response, with no value exceeding 6.0 mmol/l.

At around this time it was considered that a metabolic defect might be present, and hence samples of urine were collected from as many of the relatives as possible. Indeed, two samples were found to be positive for reducing substances, but were negative for true glucose; one also had a trace of ketones. All other urine samples were negative for all three tests.

On 09.05.73 another GTT was carried out using a loading dose of 10 g glucose. This showed an equally bizarre pattern for both the plasma glucose and 'glucose' values measured by the two methods. Moreover, the urine samples (still positive to Benedict's test) were now positive to Clinistix, with ketones being negative in all the samples.

It was by this time absolutely clear, of course, that the samples were being tampered with, but the question remained as to exactly how it was happening; hence, the next stage was to take blood from the patient in the laboratory rather than on the ward. She was, therefore, placed in a room on her own with the secretary of the department keeping a watchful eye on the situation whilst she was typing; the first four samples of a GTT were taken in the normal manner, but not leaving any bottles, etc. in the room. However, for the final half hour the door was closed and empty sample bottles were left on the bench by her side. At the appointed time blood was collected and placed in one bottle, water filled to the mark in another and the third was merely examined. The 'empty' bottle was found to contain a small amount of white powder and the other two contained high concentrations of glucose. On questioning the ward staff it then became clearer as to what might have been taking place, because in some instances it was recalled that blood and urine bottles had been left within her reach, thus giving her maximum opportunity to add powder, etc. as and whenever she wished. Probably lactose (or a lactose-containing powder) was used initially, but this was later changed to glucose.

The explanation for the supposed genetic link also became clear when it was found that the 14-year-old niece and another relative had visited their aunt in the ward that day, and that the aunt had 'volunteered' to help them label their samples. The patient was aware that a substance had been found in her own blood and urine – and of the fact that the same substance was being sought in her relatives. All relatives who had sent samples directly by post, thus 'by-passing the aunt', were negative. The diagnosis was, therefore, both Munchausen syndrome and Munchausen by proxy syndrome.

Nevertheless, Munchausen syndrome does not begin suddenly at the age of 36 years without some preceding indications – and should there be no such clues then alternative ways of finding out the past history must be sought; nor is the syndrome likely to end suddenly, either. In this case there had been three abdominal operations, one being a hysterectomy for menorrhagia and the other two being for peptic ulceration (all of which must now be regarded with some suspicion). In addition, it is of interest to document the subsequent clinical events regarding this patient.

On 07.05.73 it was noted that the right upper abdominal pain persisted, and that she had also had some bright red bleeding per rectum, although on clinical examination nothing abnormal was detected. By 12.06.73 she had realized that nobody was too concerned with her 'hyperglycaemia' and 'glycosuria'; it had previously been explained to her that 'contamination' had occurred in some way. On 07.01.75 she collapsed whilst out shopping and was taken into hospital; this episode was preceded 2 days before by a domestic upset during which her son announced that he was going to leave home. On arrival in the Accident and Emergency Department there was no evidence that she had had an epileptic fit and she regained consciousness within 3–4 h. There were comments in the case records of her responding to light, having some residual confusion, being amnesic for recent events – and there was also one view that she was merely 'sleeping'. There seemed to be generalized headache, photophobia and neck stiffness. A lumbar puncture was attempted but was unsuccessful, partly because she was so obese. She was referred to a neurosurgical unit for investigations in order to exclude a suspected subarachnoid haemorrhage; carotid angiography and a CT scan were both reported as being normal. She was ultimately returned to the hospital of origin with a diagnosis of right sided hemiparesis; on further observation the weakness of the limbs was noted to vary in degree – and even to change sides periodically. It gradually cleared up and she was able to go home, the final conclusion being that the hemiparesis was 'functional'. On 23.04.76 she presented again, with thirst, polyuria, dysuria, an eruption of boils, pruritus vulvae, and increasing weight. Very careful appraisal on this occasion truly confirmed the presence of diabetes mellitus, with the GTT being done under the strictest possible supervision!

On 17.03.77, at a time of special family problems involving her son, she was again taken to the local casualty department, this time with what she claimed to be an overdose of 1000 mg chlorpropamide, taken on the previous evening 'by mistake'. On examination she was conscious, behaving irrationally and somewhat 'hysterically'; however, the plasma glucose level was 6.0 mmol/l, thus indicating that hypoglycaemia was not the cause of her symptoms. Two months later she was accused of shoplifting; during questioning she said that she had been admitted to hospital on 15.05.77, just a few days before her arrest with hypoglycaemia on account of a chlorpropamide overdose. There was, however, no such record other than the similar story noted above and which was 2 months before. On 13.06.77 she attended the diabetic clinic, crying profusely

and asking to see a gynaecologist for her pruritus vulvae and a derma-
tologist for her boils; she had not been compliant with the therapy prescribed for her diabetes mellitus. No further details of this patient's case
history are currently available – but her imaginative presentations presumably did not end here!

In summary, much confusion was created over the years and there
were disparities galore, e.g. the high plasma 'glucose' values, the
absence of glycosuria, the positive Benedict's test on the urine, the presence of normal plasma glucose levels and the normal serum osmolality
values. Later, there was the sudden change when glycosuria appeared,
together with elevation of both plasma 'glucose' and plasma glucose, but
not the least bizarre episode was the rise and fall (of extraordinary
degree) of plasma 'glucose' in the first GTT performed. Added confusion
was caused by the positive urine tests in two relatives. It was never
established whether this lady had medical knowledge, but some information must have been available to her from some source. Moreover,
whether the positive ketones in the urine samples were caused by interference in some way was not certain.

One cannot help but think that this fantastic presentation would surely
have been one that Baron von Munchausen himself would have been
proud to have invented, and which almost certainly, therefore, would
have been included in the stories emanating from him (but written up
anonymously by Rudolf Raspe). One intriguing thought is that, had the
laboratory concerned with the original investigations already changed
over to the glucose oxidase method for routine glucose analysis, then
this patient's attempted deception might not have been detected and the
diagnosis of Munchausen syndrome would not have been made – at
least, not at that stage!

LABORATORY INVESTIGATIONS OF MUNCHAUSEN SYNDROME[104]

The diagnosis of Munchausen syndrome may be made in the chemical
pathology department of the hospital, or on account of a test result that
then permits the clinician to confirm a previous suspicion. Diuretic
compounds may be being taken in order to cause loss of weight, purgatives to produce diarrhoea and/or loss of weight, anticoagulants to precipitate haematuria and bruising, chlorpropamide to produce
hypoglycaemia, insulin to cause fits, or sleeping tablets to create

drowsiness, etc. The appropriate biochemical assays will assist in their detection. On the other hand, a patient might be contaminating biological specimens, e.g. *urine* – to which blood, lactose, glucose, organisms (from a faecal source), egg albumin (there is a different electrophoretic pattern when compared with human albumin), etc. is added; *blood* – perhaps being contaminated with glucose, lactose, etc., and *faeces* – artificially made at home and proudly presented to the outpatients department. Renal stones, supposedly passed by the patient but in reality picked up from the path on the way to the hospital, and which consequently do what no stone of biological origin ever does, namely damage the pestle and mortar used for crushing the stone prior to analysis, can be another mode of presentation of Munchausen syndrome. In this context perhaps the 'rattle test' should be added to the routine list of investigations of renal stones; this cheap test consists of simply rattling the pot in which the stone has been sent to the laboratory – the sharp sound of granite or flint on the sides of the jar is unmistakable and cannot be confused with the sound of any stone of biological origin. Faecal fat analysis, too, may provide the final clue to the diagnosis; on alkaline hydrolysis a glorious regal red colour indicates consumption of the laxative phenolphthalein – the cause of the diarrhoea that precipitated the request for the analysis in the first place!

VARIATIONS OF MUNCHAUSEN SYNDROME

In 'Munchausen syndrome by proxy' (e.g. where the mother may add substances to the child's urine in order to cause diagnostic confusion) the child may be taken into hospital for investigation. A typical feature here is that the mother is 'always' present, hardly ever leaving the child – giving an impression of utter devotion. Should narcotics be given to the child to cause drowsiness, etc. then collection of a urine sample at the appropriate time might be able to provide the information which confirms the diagnosis. There may be only a subtle difference between creating such a situation for the purpose of attention-seeking and using almost the same scenario for malicious intent.

Munchausen syndrome may not be the final diagnosis. The sequence of events may proceed to suicide (e.g. the patient who initially presents with hypoglycaemia following non-prescribed dosage with chlorpropamide and who is later found dead – perhaps from taking another pharmacological agent or through some other means); or the patient who, having taken anticoagulants to achieve attention for some reason, is found dead in a car full of exhaust fumes with a suicide note expressing great concern regarding cancer, but for which no evidence had ever been found during life – or, indeed, at postmortem examination. However, many patients with Munchausen syndrome continue to present with monotonous regularity at different clinics, in different hospitals in the country, and over a period of many years.

9
Laboratory investigations of psychiatric disorders

All the varied laboratory investigations appropriate in any clinical situation may be relevant to the diagnosis and follow-up of a psychiatric illness, especially if the mood change forms only part of the clinical presentation as a whole. Nevertheless, a great deal of clinical information, whether confirmatory, non-confirmatory or exclusory, of a particular diagnostic possibility, can be attained by performing a relatively small range of very basic tests. The tables in this chapter are intended to provide just a brief guide to some of the clinical disorders which have been alluded to in this book, together with some of the diagnoses that may be either confirmed or excluded by the tests in question (Tables 2, 3, 4)[104].

Table 2 Laboratory investigations of psychiatric disorders – urine

Procedure	Disorder
Routine procedures	
Glucose	diabetes mellitus – primary and secondary (e.g. Cushing's syndrome, phaeochromocytoma, Munchausen syndrome)
Protein	chronic renal failure, Munchausen syndrome
Ketones	diabetes mellitus, starvation, malnutrition, Munchausen syndrome
Cells	confusion in the elderly (urinary tract infection), Munchausen syndrome
Organisms	confusion in the elderly (urinary tract infection), Munchausen syndrome

Continued

Table 2 (continued)

Procedure	Disorder
Other procedures	
Electrolytes	SIADH
Osmolality	SIADH, diabetes insipidus, psychogenic polydipsia, over-enthusiastic postoperative infusion with low sodium-containing fluids
Volume (24 h)	confusion in the elderly (dehydration), diabetes insipidus, psychogenic polydipsia, over-enthusiastic postoperative infusion
Porphyrins	porphyria, hepatic disease
Porphobilinogen	porphyria
Vanillylmandelic acid (VMA)	phaeochromocytoma.
Homovanillic acid (HVA)	phaeochromocytoma
Metanephrine	phaeochromocytoma
Normetanephrine	phaeochromocytoma
Drugs	
Amphetamines	schizophrenic-like psychosis
Morphine	drug addiction
Methadone	drug addiction
Cannabis	use of cannabis
Cocaine	drug addiction
Benzodiazepines	use of benzodiazepines
Barbiturates	use of barbiturates
Codeine	use of codeine
Dihydrocodeine	use of dihydrocodeine
Heroin	drug addiction

Table 3 Laboratory investigations of psychiatric disorders – blood

Procedure	Disorder
Routine procedures	
Electrolytes and urea	Addison's disease, Cushing syndrome, diabetes mellitus, chronic renal failure, dehydration, diabetes insipidus, psychogenic polydipsia, SIADH, over-enthusiastic postoperative infusion with low sodium-containing fluids, sodium chloride ingestion
Osmolality	SIADH, Addison's disease, diabetes insipidus, psychogenic polydipsia, over-enthusiastic postoperative infusion with low sodium-containing fluids

continued

Table 3 (continued)

Procedure	Disorder
Glucose	diabetes mellitus, hypoglycaemia, Munchausen syndrome
Liver function tests	hepatitis, cirrhosis
Calcium	hyperparathyroidism (and other causes of hypercalcaemia), hypoparathyroidism (and other causes of hypocalcaemia)
γ-Glutamyl transferase	alcoholism
Full blood count (FBC)	anaemia, alcoholism (raised MCV), Munchausen syndrome (anaemia)
Prothrombin time	hepatic dysfunction, Munchausen syndrome
Other procedures	
Vitamin B_{12}	pernicious anaemia, psychosis in the elderly
Folic acid	anticonvulsant-induced neuropsychiatric symptoms, (e.g. fall of IQ, neurotic disturbance, depression, dementia, schizophrenic-like psychoses)
Ferritin	pica (e.g. pagophagia, geophagia, amylophagia, cautopyrophagia, etc.)
Alcohol	alcoholism
Cortisol	Cushing syndrome, Addison's disease
Thyroxine/TSH	hypothyroidism, hyperthyroidism, Munchausen syndrome
Insulin and C-peptide	insulinoma, Munchausen syndrome
Magnesium	severe prolonged diarrhoea, hypoparathyroidism
Lead	lead poisoning.
Adrenaline	phaeochromocytoma
Noradrenaline	phaeochromocytoma
Dexamethasone suppression test	endogenous depression
Drugs	
Lithium carbonate	monitoring lithium carbonate therapy in manic depressive psychosis (the usual aim is to achieve a serum lithium level of 0.5–0.8 mmol/l 12 h after the last dose)
Tricyclic antidepressants	validated guidelines are available for therapeutic drug monitoring (TDM) of amitriptyline, nortriptyline, imipramine, and desipramine; steady state samples are required to be taken pre-dose
Caffeine	rarely required in this context; could be used for assessing dietary intake

Table 4 Laboratory investigations of psychiatric disorders – faeces

Procedures	*Disorder*
Routine procedures	
Occult blood	Munchausen syndrome
Fat	Munchausen syndrome
Other procedures	
Phenolphthalein	Munchausen syndrome
Porphyrins	porphyria

10

Psychiatric consequences of disorders of the developing brain

with J.W.T. Dickerson

Reference has already been made to certain aspects of the developing brain. It is now necessary, however, to pursue this theme in more detail – in order to serve as background for discussion relating to those diseases where either inborn errors of metabolism or acquired metabolic disorders have psychiatric manifestations.

BRAIN DEVELOPMENT

Introduction

The CNS begins to develop very early in embryonic life. In the human, the neural plate appears down the midline of the back of the embryo during the third week following conception. Neural folds rise up on each side of the midline of the plate to form the neural tube. This tube is completed by closure at both the top and bottom ends late in the fourth week. Closure at the bottom end of the tube results in formation of the spinal cord. It is failure of the lower end to close that results in the condition known as spina bifida, a disorder now established as being related to maternal folic acid deficiency[105]. Closure at the top end of the tube results in formation of the cerebral hemispheres. Anencephaly, a condition that is incompatible with life, is failure of the brain to develop; it can result from maternal hypervitaminosis A.

Within the brain a series of overlapping phases of development characterize regional growth[106]. Expressed simply as changes in weight with time, the growth curve of the brain of man, as for all other mammalian species, follows a sigmoidal pattern[107]. The transient period of rapid developmental manifested in this curve is known as the brain growth spurt; this becomes more apparent when the growth is expressed in terms of a velocity or rate curve. In different species the growth spurt of the brain occurs at varying times with reference to a physiological milestone, such as birth. It was suggested by Davison and Dobbing[107] that the growth spurt of the brain constituted a 'critical period' when adverse influences, be they physical, metabolic or hormonal, would have their greatest effect on brain growth. The condition is complex, however, because not only anatomical and physiological but also biochemical and psychological functions of the brain have a critical period of development when they are maturing at their most rapid rates. Furthermore, the critical period of anatomical development is not the same as that for psychological development – and within each aspect of growth we also have critical periods; thus, the period of most rapid cellular division does not coincide with that for myelination or that when there is maximal dendritic arborization. There are variations, too, in different parts of the brain when, say, a particular enzyme appears or has its peak activity. In the brain, all critical periods of growth occur either during intra-uterine growth or in the early post-natal period.

Cellular growth

The nervous system contains many cell types which can broadly be categorized as neurones and glial cells. Growth of the brain occurs by either hyperplasia or hypertrophy of cells. The number of cells in the brain can be determined chemically by measuring the amount of DNA and dividing the total amount per brain, or discrete anatomical part, by the amount of DNA in a diploid nucleus (6.0 pg for man). Some tetraploid cells are present in the cortices of the cerebrum and cerebellum, but the number of these is not large enough to seriously affect the calculation. Brain tissue can also be analysed for protein and lipid; the ratio of either of these to DNA (i.e. protein/DNA or lipid/DNA) provides a measure of cell size.

For obvious reasons, rather less is known about the development of the brain of man than for other species[108]. The wet weight increases until about 6 years of age. Before birth there is a fairly linear rise in cell multiplication as indicated by accretion of DNA. Soon after birth there is a decline in DNA accretion – but synthesis continues until at least 6 years of age and possibly longer. Two peaks of DNA synthesis can be distinguished; the first of these is reached at about 18 weeks' gestation and corresponds to the maximal rate of neuronal synthesis whereas the second peak, which occurs at around birth, represents the time of most rapid glial cell division[109].

The forebrain and brain stem DNA levels attain 70% of mature values by 2 years of age, following which time they gradually increase even more to attain maximum at 6 years old. The rise of DNA in the cerebellum is more rapid, however, and achieves the adult value by 2 years. Of considerable interest is the fact that the cerebellum, comprising by weight only 10% of the whole brain, contains 30% of the total brain DNA. Post-natal growth of the cerebellum is characterized by extensive microneurone proliferation which continues up to 20 months of age. Although the control of both rate and period of DNA synthesis are largely unknown there have been suggestions that modulation of the enzymes, DNA polymerase and alkaline ribonuclease, may play a role. The increase in concentration of putrescine at the time of extensive neuronal multiplication is due to a rise in the enzyme ornithine decarboxylase, which accompanies rapid cell proliferation; the ganglioside G_{D1a}, associated with synaptic growth, also increases in the forebrain at this time.

Brain lipids

A major feature of the developing brain is the deposition of simple lipids (e.g. cholesterol) and complex lipids (e.g. phospholipids, glycolipids and other esters which contain various fatty acids). In the human the proportion of total cholesterol that is esterified in the forebrain and cerebellum falls from about 5% in early foetal life to about 1% at about 200 days' gestation; there is a small rise during early post-natal life[108]. In a number of neurological disorders, including multiple sclerosis later in life, there is an increase in cholesterol esters.

The lipid content of the human brain is fairly constant until after 7 months of gestation, following which lipid deposition increases in grey matter, reaching adult levels by 3 months post-natally. Lipid deposition in white matter continues at a more gradual rate. By 2 years of age 90% of the adult levels of lipids overall have accumulated – and by 10 years of age adult levels have been achieved.

Myelin formed around nerve axons in white matter is formed from the membranes of oligodendroglial cells; the transformation begins after these cells have ceased dividing and can be likened to a maturation process. Myelination occurs in cycles – with the process starting and proceeding to completion in different areas at different ages from late in gestation to about 30 years of age[110]. It has been estimated that myelin accounts for about 25% of the weight of the mature brain. Based on the rate of accumulation of one marker substance, namely cerebroside sulfatide, it does appear that myelin accumulates rapidly over a relatively brief period of time. Between 34 weeks and full term it rises by 300–400% and then even more rapidly between 12 and 24 weeks of age – by which time 50% of the adult amount has accumulated; the evidence is that adult levels are achieved prior to 4 years of age. It seems that the early period of myelination might play a critical role in determining whether the full adult amount will be formed. It is replication of the oligodendroglial cells, whose membranes form myelin, that is a key factor in the formation of new myelin.

The principal glycolipids in the brain are the cerebrosides and gangliosides. The latter consist of N-acetylneuraminic acid (sialic acid), sphingosine and three molecules of either glucose or galactose. A number of different gangliosides have been isolated from brain, four of these species constituting the major ones present in normal human brain; these four species together comprise 95% of the total ganglioside content. There is structural variation of the gangliosides – not only on account of the number of sialic acid molecules (i.e. mono-, di- or tri-), but also because of the actual position of sialic acid molecules within the compound (Table 5)[111]. Most of the gangliosides are located in grey matter; the greater proportion is present in dendritic and axonal complexes[112], whereas only relatively small amounts are found in the neuronal cell bodies.

One of the disialogangliosides (referred to as G_{D1a}) appears to be located specifically in dendrites and it can, therefore, be used as a quantitative measure of dendritic arborization[113]. Dendritic arborization, together with the associated process of synaptogenesis, increases slowly from 20–24 weeks' gestation – following which time there is continued increase, although at a slower rate, up to 40 weeks (full term). There then follows a considerable extension of arborization during the first 6 months after birth[106]. Experiments in rats have

Table 5 Major gangliosides of normal human brain (Svennerholm's nomenclature). From Dickerson[111]

Name	Symbol	Proposed structure
Monosialoganglioside	G_{M1}	Gal(1→3)GalNAc(1→4)Gal(1→ 4)Glu (1→1)Cer 3 ↑ 2 NeuNAC
Disialoganglioside	G_{D1a}	Gal(1→3)GalNAc(1→4)Gal(1→ 4)Glu (1→1)Cer 3 3 ↑ ↑ 2 2 NeuNAC NeuNAC
Disialoganglioside	G_{D1b}	Gal(1→3)GalNAc(1→4)Gal(1→ 4)Glu (1→1)Cer 3 ↑ 2 NeuNAC(8←2)NeuNDAC
Trisialoganglioside	G_{T1}	Gal(1→3)GalNAc(1→4)Gal(1→4)Glu (1→1)Cer 3 3 ↑ ↑ 2 2 NeuNAC NeuNAC(8⌊2)NeuNAC

Key:
Gal = galactose; GalNAc = N-acetylgalactosamine; Glu = glucose;
Cer = ceramide; NeuNAC = N-acetylneuraminic acid

confirmed that the degree of dendritic growth is affected considerably by the amount of exposure to sensory stimulation[114]. Surface glycoproteins incorporated in synaptic membranes serve as recognition factors in post-synaptic neurones; they therefore play an important role in brain function. Acetylneuraminic acid is required for synaptosomal uptake of the neurotransmitter 5HT.

Brain metabolism

Brief mention has already been made regarding the changes in brain metabolism during growth. The essential feature is that both cerebral metabolism and oxygen consumption are low at birth, but rise rapidly with growth towards maturity. At 6 years of age the brain consumes 60 ml/min of oxygen; this accounts for over half the total body basal oxygen consumption. This large amount is required in order to sustain the biosynthetic components of growth and development. Moreover, the nutrients used in sustaining oxidative metabolism also change with growth and development of the brain. Just after birth the baby is hypoglycaemic – and blood levels of ketones are also low. In normal circumstances the first food received is milk – with its relatively high fat content; this is ketogenic and there is, in consequence, a rise in blood ketone levels which continue to remain higher than at birth – up to the time of weaning. Ketones are, therefore, important fuel for the developing brain. After weaning the ketosis subsides, the enzymes essential for their metabolism also decrease and glucose then becomes the major energy substrate. In the mature brain the metabolism of ketones is limited by permeability; moreover, the permeability characteristics vary from region to region within the brain depending on the nature of the blood–brain barrier. It is well recognized that in the neonate this barrier is under-developed, so that regional differences do not occur.

Much of the glucose used in the brain in early life is metabolized by way of the hexose monophosphate shunt. The neonatal brain will withstand hypoxia for a longer period of time than the adult brain. This probably reflects the predominance of glycolysis during early brain development. After birth respiration becomes increasingly important until it assumes the dominant role in glucose metabolism. The brain uses the carbon skeleton from glucose metabolism to make glutamate and aspartate (Figure 9)[108]. Alanine is derived from pyruvate by transamination, glutamine from glutamate by amidation and aminobutyrate from glutamate by decarboxylation.

The unique importance of glucose metabolism in the adult brain is partly due to the blood–brain barrier. The high rate of influx of amino acids into the neonatal brain is thought to be due to absence of the barrier at this phase of development; later, amino acid transport mechanisms develop within the barrier. Each of these mechanisms permits transport of a specific group of amino acids to meet the demand of the brain for that group, entirely independent of the other systems. It is now known that there are three separate, saturable stereospecific transport systems, these being for neutral, basic and acidic amino acids, respectively. Within each group of amino acids there is competition so that transport of one member of a group is competitively inhibited by the others of that group. This is well

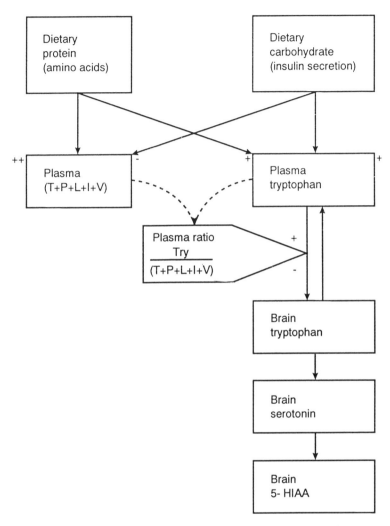

Figure 18 Dietary protein and carbohydrate in the control of brain serotonin synthesis

illustrated by the competition that exists between tryptophan and the other LNAA. The transport of tryptophan into the brain, and hence the synthesis of 5HT, is determined by the secretion of insulin which also facilitates the passage of the competing amino acids into muscle, thus reducing their concentration in plasma and increasing the tryptophan : LNAA ratio (Figure 18)[113,115,116].

179

The active processes in the blood–brain barrier are very susceptible to both oxygen supply and metabolic inhibitors. Although the amino acids entering the brain are used for protein synthesis there are some, which in their own right, are neurotransmitters; yet others are precursors of neurotransmitters. Many brain proteins are being formed continuously throughout life, even within the diurnal rhythm of a single day. The complexity of proteins in the brain makes it impossible to even consider a 'critical' or 'vulnerable' period in brain protein development.

PSYCHIATRIC IMPLICATIONS OF DISORDERS OF THE DEVELOPING BRAIN

In childhood there can occur, from time to time – and in a similar manner to those individuals who possess a fully mature nervous system (already discussed in detail in the previous chapter) – various forms of psychological problems and frank psychiatric presentations. When considering the developing brain it is necessary, however, to recognize one further category of disorder, namely that of mental retardation. In keeping with the title of this volume, it is only those conditions with an important chemical/biochemical cause that are documented here. In this context, therefore, mental retardation is divided into those which have either an inherited or an acquired metabolic basis.

Hence, in the latter portion of this chapter there will be detailed reference to each of these three categories of disorder in which chemical/biochemical derangements are either causal or contributory to the mental state; there will be sections on selected 'inherited metabolic disorders', some 'acquired metabolic disorders' and other incidental chemical, biochemical, pharmacological and toxicological causes of 'psychological/psychiatric disorders in neonatal life, infancy and childhood'.

Mental retardation – inherited and acquired[91,117]

Many mentally retarded patients have clinical evidence of an 'early occurring' or a 'later manifesting' inherited biochemical disturbance. Such disorders can be classified according to their aetiology, associated biochemical disturbances, principal metabolic features or clinical expression; a large number of these disorders have been reviewed recently in considerable detail[97] and for this reason only a few selected examples will be discussed here. Some of the more frequently seen mental abnormalities with a biochemical basis include the amino-acidurias and organic acidurias, together with hormonal, lysosomal, mitochondrial and peroxisomal disorders, although there are, in fact, many other inherited errors of metabolism that present in a similar way.

Many determinants for mental retardation as a whole have now been identified – including the preconceptual disorders (e.g. inborn errors of metabolism). However, not all cases of mental retardation are genetically determined, some being secondary to various causes or events; there can be, for instance early embryonic disruption (e.g. due to chromosomal disorders, infections and exposure to teratogens) and some occur on account of various provocations to which the foetal brain is prone (e.g. infections and toxins). To this list must be added the consequences of perinatal difficulties (e.g. prematurity, hypoxia, hypoglycaemia, hyperbilirubinaemia and infections) and other insults to which the postnatal brain is subject (e.g. infections, asphyxia, hypo-glycaemia, hypernatraemia, toxins and malnutrition)[118].

Environmental and psychosocial factors

Besides the genetically based causes of mental retardation – and the large number of acquired conditions, there are other very different disorders in which one or more of a multitude of environmental factors (physical, biological, psychological or social) is/are responsible for determining the clinical presentation. It should be appreciated, moreover, that some or all of these environmental factors – most of them variable in nature, in degree and in timing – could either singly or collectively also contribute to the modification of an already established case of mental retardation.

Psychosocial factors are just one special group of environmental determinants influencing mental function. Any of the many miscellaneous psychosocial circumstances (e.g. family organizational problems and psychopathology within the parents) must be taken into consideration when attempting to assess children with later occurring psychiatric problems (Table 6). Subcultural mental retardation is largely confined to social class V of the population; it is clearly best represented in the poorer areas of large towns and cities, where economic problems thrive – and also within problem families where there might be poverty, debt, lack of good education, poor nutrition and deprivation of proper care. These factors are referred to because they will contribute, perhaps in a small or large way, to the final state of mind. It is important to remember that clinical consequences of the actual timing of deprivation of environmental stimulation or emotion is just as important as observing the timing of intrusions such as biological insults (e.g. infections, drugs, metabolic factors, etc.) when seeking to determine the probable course of events during the course of an illness. The final mental outcome in all of us must surely be a very complex function of the intricate interactions between all the components of this vast assembly of protean factors/situations.

INHERITED METABOLIC DISORDERS

As referred to earlier, there are many inborn errors of metabolism which, for various reasons, lead to impaired functioning or development of the brain; some cause irreversible lesions and are permanent, whereas others are frankly progressive. Some of these disorders, however, are remediable by therapeutic or dietary intervention, provided firstly that diagnosis is made soon after birth when the brain is still growing and developing at a rapid rate, and secondly that management begins without undue delay. These latter conditions are, therefore, of particular importance clinically; accordingly, some of them feature in the selection of inherited presentations which are dealt with briefly in this section.

Congenital primary hypothyroidism[119]

Clinical aspects

Recognition that a postmature, large baby, with a wide posterior fontanelle, an umbilical hernia and a goitre might have congenital hypothyroidism is the earliest clinical way of being alerted to the possibility of this diagnosis; there may well also be delayed bone age.

The early signs that might be found in the first 4 weeks of life are that the infant is placid and sleepy; there may also be prolongation of 'physiological' jaundice, a history of poor feeding, constipation and abdominal distension. Later, the appearance is more obviously cretinous, with a tongue that is large, a hoarse cry, and skin and hair that both look and feel dry; the responses are slow and there is a failure of growth. Retarded development, both physical and mental, is characteristic. In the absence of treatment an IQ of 80 or less is probable.

The commonest and most important cause of congenital hypothyroidism is thyroid dysgenesis, in which there is an association with Down syndrome; it is a sporadic condition with a frequency of about 1 in 3500 births, is of unknown aetiology and 65% of the cases are female. Approximately 65% of infants possess some thyroid tissue and when such cases are studied overall there is revealed to be a spectrum of degrees of hypothyroidism. The second most common cause of congenital hypothyroidism, accounting for approximately 15% of those cases identified by the screening of newborn babies, is dyshormonogenesis. These cases are recessively inherited disorders of the various enzymes involved in iodothyronine synthesis. In addition, there are less common causes such as those where the condition is secondary to pituitary or hypothalamic problems. Moreover, during the process of attempting to establish the correct diagnosis, consideration must be given to the possibility of there being one of the transient disorders of thyroid function – of which there are several types. It should be remembered that maternal antithyroid drug administration, given in the second and third trimester of pregnancy for the treatment of thyrotoxicosis, is a cause of hypothyroidism and goitre in the newborn infant.

Biochemical basis

The incidence of congenital hypothyroidism is approximately 1 in 3000 births. It is important to diagnose the disorder as soon as possible because delay in the institution of therapy will lead to a poor intellectual and neurological prognosis. The manifestations of hypothyroidism steadily progress in the absence of treatment and attain full physical and mental expression by about 3–6 months of age, unless the metabolic defect is only partial, in which case onset of presentation is delayed, symptoms are milder and the syndrome as a whole is incomplete. Thyroid hormone deficiency leads to retarded brain growth and defective myelination, together with adverse effects on cell acquisition, dendritic arborization, synaptic organization and maturation of neurotransmitter systems[91]. Should replacement therapy not be adequate then, as already stated, intellectual development is likely to be suboptimal.

Phenylketonuria (PKU)[120]

Clinical aspects

Many different conditions causing elevation of blood phenylalanine levels (hyperphenylalaninaemia) are detected by the screening procedure as applied to the blood of newborn babies. The most important of these is phenylketonuria which is caused by deficiency of the enzyme phenylalanine hydroxylase. The classical presentation is of an infant with fair hair, blue eyes and, if untreated, mental retardation, with an IQ of less than 50; there may also be seizures and eczema. The other conditions need to be excluded before long-term dietary management is instituted; early diagnosis permits a better prognosis than would be obtained from commencing correct management after onset of symptoms. Nevertheless, it does seem from recent observations made on unaffected siblings that mild intellectual deficit is the likely outcome; recommendations as regards dietary management are now being tightened in order to avoid this and other late onset neurological abnormalities. In order to avoid serious foetal consequences it is vital to ensure that the maternal diet is strictly adhered to – from prior to the time of conception.

Biochemical basis

Phenylketonuria, the most common genetically determined amino acid disorder in Caucasians, is of autosomal recessive inheritance; heterozygotes are free of symptoms. Deficiency of phenylalanine hydroxylase is the cause. It occurs in approximately 1 in 10 000 births. High concentrations of phenylalanine interfere with the processes of myelination, protein synthesis and the entry of other essential amino acids to the brain; high concentrations of phenylalanine metabolites have been shown *in vitro* to inhibit some of the enzymes involved in glycolysis and pyruvate metabolism and to also interfere with neurotransmitter synthesis.

Hartnup disease[121]

Clinical aspects

In most cases the children with this abnormality, identified by routine urine screening, do not seem to suffer any clinical abnormality at all. In some cases, however, cutaneous photosensitivity is seen, with the skin becoming red and roughened after just moderate exposure to the sun. Should exposure be more prolonged then a pellagra-like rash, pruritus and eczema may appear. Although the first case described in the literature was accompanied by mental deficiency this has not occurred in other patients. However, psychological features may be seen periodically in some individuals, interspaced with long periods of spontaneous remission. The features comprise irritability, emotional instability, confusion and suicidal tendancies; all being linked more often than not to reversible cerebellar ataxic episodes, some of which are accompanied by a skin rash as described above.

Biochemical basis

Hartnup disease, named after the first patient described, is one of the commonest inherited disorders of amino acids and is of autosomal recessive inheritance; it occurs in approximately 1 in 24000 births. There is increased urinary output of neutral urinary amino acids (monoamino-monocarboxylic amino acids); these comprise alanine, serine, threonine, valine, leucine, isoleucine, phenylalanine, tyrosine, tryptophan and histidine, whereas proline, hydroxyproline and arginine remain normal. This observation is important in distinguishing the condition from Fanconi syndrome in which the aminoaciduria is generalized and not selective. The serum amino acids are not elevated in Hartnup disease, which is due to a single defect, in both the intestinal mucosa and renal tubules involving the transport of neutral amino acids.

The nicotinic acid need of the body is met in part by endogenous synthesis from tryptophan, although some comes from direct dietary intake. In this context it is important to observe that one of the amino acids that is poorly absorbed from the intestine in Hartnup disease is tryptophan; the unfortunate consequence is that depletion of nicotinic acid, which leads to pellagra, can follow. Nicotinic acid is the precursor of nicotinamide which is a component of the coenzymes NAD and NADP; these two coenzymes are, in turn, essential for the efficient working of two particularly important biochemical processes – glycolysis and oxidative phosphorylation.

Galactosaemia[91,120]

Clinical aspects

This condition usually presents acutely within the first week of life with lethargy and vomiting; progression is rapid and by the end of the week the illness is usually life-threatening with hepatic necrosis and possibly septicaemia. In most cases the disease will terminate in death if it remains undiagnosed and untreated. Nevertheless, in some individuals the condition is milder, in which case the presentation is one of cataracts and mental retardation with an IQ often in the range of 60–80; this equates with learning difficulties. In a few cases the condition does not cause symptoms and the intellect remains good. In general, the response to dietary withdrawal of galactose in the acute stage is life saving, but even those who are promptly so treated often end up with an intellectual deficit with possible neurological signs too. Even in those who attain normal intelligence it is not uncommon to find significant behavioural and emotional disturbance.

Biochemical basis

The incidence of galactosaemia is approximately 1 in 60 000 births. It is the enzyme galactose-1-phosphate uridyl transferase that is deficient in this disorder; in consequence there is intracellular accumulation of the highly toxic galactose-1-phosphate. It is genetically transmitted as an autosomal recessive characteristic. Several factors may be involved in the development of the neurological deficit here and additional forces may operate at around the perinatal period when cerebral oedema may be the result of hepatic and renal dysfunction. Amongst a number of biochemical abnormalities found within brain tissue in this disorder, it has been found that there is reduction both in cerebrosides and protein-bound hexosamine.

Homocystinuria[122]

Clinical aspects

Infants with homocystinuria Type I are normal at birth. During infancy nonspecific symptoms develop, including failure to thrive and consequential delay in development. Subluxation of the lens of the eye (ectopia lentis) is not usually recognized until the child is over three years of age, at which time myopia and quivering of the iris is observed. Later in life other ophthalmological problems ensue in the form of astigmatism, glaucoma and cataracts and perhaps also optic atrophy and detachment of the retina. A wide variety of skeletal abnormalities can be found in these patients and although some do retain normal intelligence there are many who display mental retardation. In addition, more than half of those with the condition develop various psychiatric disorders. In this context it is important to be aware that thromboembolic episodes commonly occur in large and small blood vessels anywhere in the body but particularly in the brain. It is recommended that all these patients are given a special diet restricted in methionine but supplemented with cysteine, together with medication in the form of a high dose of vitamin B_6 with the addition of folic acid if vitamin B_6 alone does not cause dramatic improvement.

Biochemical basis

Homocysteine, not normally detected in normal serum or urine, is an intermediate compound of methionine degradation, which is normally remethylated to methionine. Three variants of the disorder have been identified, each of them being biochemically subtly different. They are referred to as homocystinuria Types I, II, and III. Homocystinuria Type I is the commonest variant and occurs in approximately 1 in 200000 births. It is transmitted as an autosomal recessive condition. There is elevation of both methionine and homocystine in body fluids but it is important to know that only fresh urine should be analysed for homo-cystine as the compound is degraded in urine that is stored.

Maple syrup urine disease (MSUD)[123]

Clinical aspects

In the classic form of maple syrup disease the infant is normal at birth, but in the first week of life poor feeding is noted and vomiting occurs. Neurological signs soon develop and there is alternating hypertonicity and flaccidity; convulsions also feature and hypoglycaemia is common, although correcting this does not lead to improvement of the clinical presentation. It is common for there to be both mental and neurological consequences. If the disorder is not treated then death will occur within the first few months. There are synthetic foods available in which leucine, isoleucine and valine are not present and which must be consumed for the rest of life.

Biochemical basis

The name given to this disease is simply based on the fact that the odour of the urine is indistinguishable from that of fresh maple syrup; indeed, it is not only the urine that has this odour but also the sweat and cerumen. There is marked elevation in both urine and serum of leucine, isoleucine and valine. Several varieties of the disorder exist; all are transmitted as an autosomal recessive trait. The incidence is of the order of 1 in 250 000 births, although in the United States the Mennon-ites have a higher incidence of the classic form of the disease.

Menkes' kinky hair syndrome[124]

Clinical aspects

Within a few weeks of birth drowsiness and lethargy appear, together with feeding difficulties. Progressive mental retardation invariably follows. The appearance of the hair is characteristic; it becomes depigmented, develops a coarse feel and there is less of it. Death usually occurs by the age of 10 years.

Biochemical basis

In this X-linked recessive disorder serum copper and caeruloplasmin levels are low; gut and kidney copper is increased, although brain and liver copper is decreased. The incidence is approximately 1 in 255000 births. There is cerebral and cerebellar degeneration and the brain is small. The copper-containing enzymes lysyl oxidase, dopamine β-hydroxylase, tyrosinase and superoxide dismutase are all functionally impaired and probably underlie, at least in part, clinical expression of the disease. The location of the Menkes gene is now known precisely; it codes for a protein which is homologous with membrane-bound cation-transporting adenosine triphosphatase (ATPase) proteins.

Wilson's disease (hepatolenticular degeneration)[125]

Clinical aspects

Wilson's disease may present in childhood or later in adult life. Should it present early in life there is likely to be haemolytic anaemia or a hepatic problem (hepatitis or cirrhosis) but if it manifests later then a neurological disorder (with progressive extrapyramidal signs and symptoms) may be dominant, although this would usually be in association with hepatic dysfunction. A Kayser–Fleischer ring is found around the corneal limbus and forms after the first decade; this may only be detectable by means of slit-lamp examination in children and comprises copper deposited in Descemet's membrane. Approximately 20% of cases present with either a psychiatric or a behavioural disturbance, any of which could antedate or even occur simultaneously with one of the other presentations. An extremely wide variety of mental abnormalities can be identified in patients with Wilson's disease; they range from change of personality, emotional disturbance, deterioration in school performance, cognitive impairment, frank psychoses, to progressive dementia. The patient may express irritability, anxiety, emotional lability, euphoria, excitement, rage, violence, and 'hysteria', but can sometimes be withdrawn – displaying apathy and depression. Psychoses seen during the course of Wilson's disease include schizophrenia with hallucinations, hypomania and depression. These are not necessarily of long duration and can sometimes occur transiently. The extrapyramidal features are responsible for the deterioration of handwriting that may be seen at some stage of the disorder.

Biochemical basis

The basic biochemical disturbance in this condition is disordered copper metabolism. The serum copper is normally low (although in hepatic failure the level may be markedly raised on account of its release from the liver) and the caeruloplasmin value is decreased, although it may be at the lower end of the reference range should there be an accompanying acute-phase reaction (i.e. caeruloplasmin is one of many acute-phase reactants which rise in the presence of inflammation). Deposition of copper in various parts of the brain is fundamental to both CNS and psychological expressions of the disease. Urine and liver copper levels are increased. The incidence is of the order of 1 in 500 000 births; it is of autosomal recessive inheritance.

Lysosomal storage disorders[126]

Clinical aspects

The mode of clinical expression of the large number of disorders in this category of diseases varies widely; mental retardation and neurological abnormalities feature highly. However, in some of the diseases there is involvement of tissues other than the brain, e.g. bone, liver, heart or skin, and not all of them are associated with mental retardation. Hence, many of the disorders present with special identifying features; moreover, the various disorders present at different ages, although most are expressed overtly in early paediatric life. The principal feature of the majority of conditions, however, is that they cause mental retardation on account of deposition of complex lipids within the neuronal cells. In these cases the infant is initially clinically normal but sooner or later develops signs of slowing of development. There then follows gradual progressive loss of the abilities previously gained, moving towards the point of inanition and terminal respiratory infection. Some of the diseases progress at a much slower pace than others, however, thus accounting for the very great variations that are possible in clinical presentation. It is possible to classify these diseases broadly into the following groups – the lipidoses, the mucopolysaccharidoses, the glycoproteinoses, the mucolipidoses and a few other miscellaneous conditions. Names linked with some of the mucopolycaccharidoses include Hurler, Scheie, Hurler–Scheie, Hunter, Sanfilippo, Morquio and Maroteaux. Many of these conditions have now been divided into several sub-types on biochemical grounds. The lipidoses include G_{M1}-gangliosidosis, G_{M2}-gangliosidosis (Tay–Sachs disease), G_{M2}-gangliosidosis (Sandhoff disease), metachromatic leucodystrophy, Gaucher's disease, Niemann–Pick disease, Fabry disease, Krabbe disease, Farber disease, and Wolman's disease.

Biochemical basis

Complex molecules such as proteins, glycoproteins, glycolipids and proteoglycans, are found in all body tissues; they are catabolized by the degradatory enzymes within the lysosomes, which are intracellular organelles lying within the membranes of cells. Should any of these enzymes be deficient then a metabolic blockage will occur thus causing excessive accumulation of the substance that would normally have been changed in that biochemical reaction. Each clinical disorder referred to above is accounted for by deficiency of a different enzyme in the metabolic pathway. In Tay–Sachs disease, for example, electron microscopy reveals the neuronal protoplasm to be crowded with large numbers of ovoid membranous bodies caused by the accumulation of lipids in layers. Most of the lysosomal disorders are of autosomal inheritance, although both Hunter and Fabry diseases are transmitted by X-linked inheritance. The approximate incidence of these disorders grouped as a whole is similar to that of phenylketonuria. However, the incidence of one specific example, e.g. the late infantile form of metachromatic leucodystrophy, is about 1 in 40000 births; Tay–Sachs disease occurs in approximately 1 in 3000 births among Ashkenazi Jews.

ACQUIRED METABOLIC DISORDERS

Developmental abnormalities of the nervous system in which there are mental consequences can be attributed to a number of causes. These include certain chromosomal anomalies, a variety of infections, exposure to teratogens, maternal nutritional deficiencies and excesses, exposure of the growing foetus to an abnormal chemical environment (e.g. treated, untreated or inadequately controlled maternal disease) and some disorders of multiple aetiology in which various non-specific defects of embryogenesis are basic to the clinical presentation. It is only those disorders in which there has been some definite chemical/biochemical association that will be elaborated upon in this section. In particular, it is those situations where there has been known exposure to teratogens during the course of pregnancy, or even antecedent to it should there have been cumulation of the agent in question, that will receive special attention here. The principle disorders of intra-uterine and maternal origin are detailed below. Disorders occurring later – at the time of birth, neonatally, postnatally and during childhood are considered in the section entitled 'Disorders in neonatal life, infancy and childhood' (p. 198).

Foetal alcohol syndrome[127–132]

Clinical aspects

Maternal alcohol consumption is claimed to be the most common single cause of mental handicap and there is often associated growth retardation. Two drinks a day, or approximately 100 ml alcohol per week, is known to produce measurable restriction of growth together with increased foetal loss; smaller amounts of alcohol can produce milder abnormalities. Maternal intake of 90 ml of alcohol a day can be regarded as a major risk to the infant[131,132]. Nevertheless, the female response to alcohol is so varied, with some women responding much more sensitively than others. Although only a small percentage of foetuses so exposed express the syndrome, the only safe advice to those who are pregnant is to recommend taking no alcohol at all as no safe limit in pregnancy has been established. The time of critical exposure seems to be prior to the eighth week of intra-uterine life; indeed, it is well established that consumption of alcohol during the first four weeks after conception can be associated with a multitude of craniofacial abnormalities. The consequences for the baby of alcohol consumption by the mother include alcohol withdrawal in the immediate postnatal period – expressed in the form of tremulousness, hyperactivity and irritability. However, the tremulousness is sometimes of much longer duration than would be generally expected, the irritability might extend into infancy, even later there may be hyperkinesis and moreover, permanent fine motor dysfunction can sometimes remain. There may also be mental retardation with a mean IQ of around 60–70. Alcohol ingestion leads not only to an increased foetal loss rate but also to a high perinatal death rate.

Biochemical basis

The pathogenesis of mental retardation, the psychological changes, neurological features, craniofacial abnormalities and growth retardation consequent on alcohol consumption is at present conjectural, although a number of hypotheses have been advanced. It is possible that it is interaction with nutrients that is the basis; in this context it is known that there are a number of specific nutritional deficiencies characteristic of alcoholics including those of vitamin A, folic acid, zinc and magnesium. Protein-energy malnutrition may play a part. Alternatively, it could be that there is true toxicity from the alcohol itself from formation of acetaldehyde in the placenta. Moreover, intake of alcohol and the smoking of tobacco are commonly associated and it is possible that synergism between the two could be important.

Maternal exposure to pharmacological agents and various chemicals[129,133]

Clinical aspects

Medication with either aminopterin or methotrexate over the period from 4–10 weeks of gestation has been associated with hydrocephalus or anencephaly. Warfarin given during the second or third trimester of pregnancy is reported to cause microcephaly and mental retardation. Methyl mercury intoxication in the mother leads to microcephaly and mental retardation, and vitamin A or retinoic acid derivatives in high doses can produce hydrocephalus and/or microcephaly. Phenytoin administration has been associated with microcephaly and mental retardation in a small percentage of foetuses so exposed and, exactly as in the case of alcohol, no safe dose has been established. Another drug with antiepileptic activity is sodium valproate; if taken during the course of pregnancy there is found to be an association with open spina bifida[134]. In addition, most of the compounds quoted above can also cause other foetal malformations of a more minor nature. Malformations of the central nervous system can be caused by medications such as troxidone and bromides; there can also be similar consequences from taking many of the various drugs of addiction, including heroin and cocaine and so too with the organic solvents and polychlorinated biphenyls.

As in the case of anticonvulsants, the continuation of long-term psychotropic medication during pregnancy raises difficult clinical issues. Risk–benefit consideration, both for the foetus and the mother, have to be carefully assessed. In the case of antipsychotic medication for example, extrapyramidal symptoms in the neonate have occasionally been reported. Similarly, there have been some cases of lithium toxicity and neonatal goitre when maternal therapy was not carefully monitored. Although teratogenic effects of antidepressants are probably very rare, the manufacturers of sertraline (an SSRI antidepressant) have advised extra caution in its use during pregnancy.

Biochemical basis

A number of drugs taken during the course of pregnancy are known to cause foetal malformations and/or mental sequelae. For this reason it is generally considered inadvisable to take any drug or compound at this time unless it is well proven that it is safe to do so. Factors that may affect the outcome include the dose given, the frequency of administration, the stage of pregnancy, duration of medication, susceptibility of the individual to drug toxicity, maternal nutritional status and any variability that might exist for any reason in maternal metabolism.

In general, it seems that drugs given to the mother in the 2 weeks after conception either cause foetal death or have no consequence at all. Drugs given during the rest of the first trimester might cause congenital malformations and drugs given in the second and third trimesters may have adverse effects on growth and development[133]. There is evidence that the foetal ability to metabolize exogenous biological substances is excellent; a problem is more likely to arise from the frequency with which the mother takes certain medications. Should there be just a small number of doses, or perhaps only a single dose of a rapidly cleared compound, then very little will reach the foetus. A more serious problem would arise if the foetus suffered high drug exposure on account of regular and repeated maternal dosing[133].

In the introduction to the section on brain development at the beginning of this chapter, reference was made to maternal folic acid deficiency causing spina bifida. In this context it should be noted that anticonvulsant drugs, such as phenytoin and phenobarbitone, induce biochemical evidence of folate deficiency in those who are already nutritionally deficient or borderline in their daily intake. With reference to the psychotropic drugs discussed above, it is established that they too can cause folate deficiency.

Maternal iodine deficiency[135–137]

Clinical aspects

It has long been established that iodine deficiency can cause mental retardation and other clinical sequelae of thyroid insufficiency in geographic areas where endemic goitres occur. This endemic form of cretinism is divisible into two syndromes – namely the 'nervous syndrome' and the 'myxoedematous syndrome'. The former is characterized by mental retardation and other CNS features; the evidence from Papua New Guinea is that iodine deficiency itself, in the first trimester of pregnancy (i.e. before development of the foetal thyroid gland) has damaged the developing nervous system, quite apart from any effect it may have on thyroid hormone synthesis. In the latter syndrome there is mental retardation with myxoedema but no overt CNS problems; the iodine deficiency in this case comes much later, in late foetal life and during the postnatal period.

Biochemical basis

The normal dietary intake of iodine is approximately $250\,\mu g/d$, although additional iodine for thyroid hormone biosynthesis comes from iodized salt and iodate in bread. In addition, a further supply is made available from the metabolism of thyroid hormones. Even if the intake of iodine is small the iodide trapping mechanism within the thyroid gland is a very efficient process. However, in geographic areas where the intake of iodine is less than $60\,\mu g/d$ clinically obvious goitres are commonly found. Should the intake be less than 20 μg/d goitres may be very large indeed and, on account of compensatory mechanisms being incomplete, endemic cretinism can arise.

Maternal phenylketonuria (PKU)[138–141]

Clinical aspects

Inadequately controlled maternal phenylketonuria can cause mental retardation, microcephaly, other CNS signs, congenital heart defects and intrauterine growth retardation (IUGR) in the nonphenylketonuric offspring. There is, in addition, a greater risk of spontaneous abortion. It is essential to commence a restricted phenylalanine intake prior to conception, as this is the only way to produce a satisfactory outcome[138,139,141].

Biochemical basis

The basis is that the brain cells of the nonphenylketonuric foetus are exposed to excessive quantities of phenylalanine, in analogous manner to exposure of the newborn baby with PKU to the same amino acid in high amounts postnatally. There is, however, observed to be greater sensitivity in foetal life because phenylalanine levels which are known to be safe postnatally can produce damage during the developmental phase (Table 6)[141].

Table 6 Maternal phenylalaninaemia: risk of damage to foetus according to maternal phenylalanine level (reproduced with permission from Campbell, A.G.M. and McIntosh, N. (1992). *Forfar and Arneil's Textbook of Paediatrics*, Churchill Livingstone)

	Blood phenylalanine (mmol/l)		
	>1.25	0.65–1.2	< 0.625
Spontaneous abortion (%)	24	22	8
Mental retardation (%)	92	53	21
Microencephaly (%)	73	57	24
Congenital heart disease (%)	12	11	0
Low birthweight (%)	40	52	13

Maternal zinc deficiency

Clinical aspects

Maternal dietary zinc deficiency may have profound effects on the outcome of pregnancy. In this context it is during the last trimester that approximately 65% of the total zinc needed by the foetus is actually utilised. There is evidence that if the maternal diet is poor in protein then the mother's total body zinc will be low; the latter, in turn, is the direct cause of the foetal zinc stores becoming depleted and this leads ultimately to foetal growth retardation. From studies on small-for-dates infants (SFD) there are also indications that the function of the CNS may be permanently impaired in that large numbers of such children are found to have low IQ scores, poor school performance and behavioural problems, together with other signs of minimal brain damage[142,143]. However, a study of infants subjected to prenatal undernutrition as a result of the famine in Holland in the Second World War showed that the infants had normal mental functioning later in life[144]. The implied recovery in this situation may have been influenced by a good environment into which the babies were born.

In a study of small for gestational age (SGA) babies, with birth weights of 2.0 SD or more below the mean, it was confirmed at the postmortem examinations that growth retardation affected all organs of the body to varying degrees. The brain, however, was least affected in these asymmetrically growth retarded infants who were observed to have relatively large heads[145]. Nevertheless, some babies are found to have equal reduction in both brain and body and they are referred to as being symmetrically growth retarded. They are normal small babies who have low birth weights, not because of true growth retardation but simply on account of low genetic growth potential. On the whole, the evidence is that slow intrauterine growth affects the brain less than might be expected although there are some especially vulnerable periods during gestation. Neuronal cell multiplication occurs at around 10–18 weeks of gestation, in the first trimester of pregnancy, and it is at this time that adverse factors affecting the foetus might cause subsequent microcephaly. As the neuronal cells grow they develop dendritic processes and then synaptic connections. It is not until the second trimester that glial cells commence multiplying, but they continue to do so after birth during the growth spurt phase[145,146]. It seems that prolonged slow head growth from early on in the second trimester of pregnancy predisposes the infant to a higher incidence of clumsiness, difficulty with learning and disturbance of behaviour, perhaps due to hypoxia and hypoglycaemia *in utero*[147].

Biochemical basis

During pregnancy, maternal leucocyte zinc concentration normally falls on account of hormonal influences; a greater than normal fall occurs in association with IUGR[148,149]. Physiologically, iron competes with zinc for the same absorptive mechanism and hence, if iron supplements are given during a pregnancy in which zinc status has been of border-line adequacy, zinc deficiency may be thereby induced.

DISORDERS IN NEONATAL LIFE, INFANCY AND CHILDHOOD

In this section only specific paediatric problems will be presented. It must be remembered, of course, that from time to time many of the disorders seen later in life and already discussed in the previous chapter, might also occur at this younger age.

Hypocalcaemia[119]

Clinical aspects

Presenting features in an infant with hypocalcaemia include irritability, twitching, tremors and seizures. Some infants, however, display lethargy, vomiting and difficulties with feeding. The traditional signs that are used later in life – namely the Chvostek and Trousseau signs – are not reliable in the newborn baby. However, there is prolongation of the QT interval on the ECG and there is a risk of sudden cardiac death. Neonatal hypocalcaemia can appear early or late. Should the hypocalcaemia occur early, i.e. during the first three days of life, then it is usual for it to resolve spontaneously within a few days. However, symptomatic hypocalcaemia is seen more frequently in preterm babies where the ability to secrete PTH in response to hypocalcaemia is impaired. It also occurs in babies born to mothers with diabetes mellitus, where there has been asphyxia at birth and where there has been any other cause of perinatal stress. Late neonatal hypocalcaemia is not as common as it used to be; it presented around the fifth to the seventh day of life in normal term infants and was due to the high phosphate and low calcium content of unmodified cow's milk leading to hyperphosphataemia which, in turn, caused hypocalcaemia. Hypomagnesaemia can itself cause hypocalcaemia because it inhibits PTH secretion; moreover, depletion of magnesium also diminishes tissue response to any PTH that is released. Hypoparathyroidism is another well recognized cause of low serum calcium. If the mother has hypercalcaemia for any reason then the foetal parathyroid glands become suppressed; nevertheless, the neonatal hypocalcaemia that results usually resolves spontaneously. In addition, alkalosis leads to hypocalcaemia.

Biochemical basis

A neonate with a serum total calcium of less than 1.75 mmol/l would be regarded as having hypocalcaemia. Earlier reference (Chapter 5) has been made to the vital role of calcium in the processes of neural transmission, nerve excitability and neurotransmitter secretion – all being basic to the clinical expressions described above.

Hypoglycaemia[150,151]

Clinical aspects

Hypoglycaemia is a common cause of a baby being jittery or floppy. Other expressions of hypoglycaemia include tremor, hypotonia, an abnormal cry and irritability. There may also be feeding difficulties, convulsions, coma or even sudden death. However, it is also well recognized that profound hypoglycaemia may occur in the absence of any obvious clinical manifestations.

Transient hypoglycaemia can occur in the neonate on account of decreased production of glucose (e.g. due to prematurity, birth asphyxia, starvation or sepsis) but it also occurs in babies that are small in relation to gestational age, due to low liver glycogen deposits. In normal circumstances glycogen deposition in the liver is largely a function of the third trimester of pregnancy. Transient hypoglycaemia also occurs where there is hyperinsulinism of short duration which thereby leads to an increased rate of disappearance of glucose (e.g. as happens in the infant of a mother with diabetes mellitus, or where there has been maternal glucose infusion). Hypoglycaemia may, on the other hand, be persistent or recurrent; in this case there may be persistent hyperinsulinism with increased utilization of glucose (e.g. an insulin secreting adenoma, etc.) or possibly decreased production of glucose, as occurs with hormone deficiencies (e.g. glucagon or cortisol) and occasionally in hypopituitarism. Some of the inborn errors of metabolism also cause lessened production of glucose[150].

Biochemical basis

The glucose need of the brain of a newborn infant is around 5.5 mg/kg/min; this compares with the requirement of the brain of a 6-year-old child of greater than 3.0 mg/kg/min. These figures equate with approximately 60–80% of the daily output by the liver of glucose. It is not difficult to see why hypoglycaemia ranks as an important paediatric problem. Although it is commonly known that moderate hypoglycaemia can cause behavioural changes, it is important to emphasise that more severe and prolonged depletion of glucose can lead to neurological damage which is permanent.

Hypoxia[152–156]

Clinical aspects

Hypoxia, consequent on the complications that can sometimes occur in the premature infant and in the neonate, has long been regarded as being causal of subsequent hyperactivity, impulsivity, difficulties in socialization and poor control of emotions – especially anger. However, there is some controversy over these beliefs and they do not receive the full support of all clinical investigators[152,153].

Inadequate oxygenation of the foetus is the major cause of perinatal death and disability; it is the brain and heart tissues that are especially prone to suffer hypoxic damage. The principal clinical presentations of hypoxia in the newborn infant are based, in sequence of appearance, on antepartum hypoxia, intrapartum hypoxia, postnatal hypoxia and the hypoxia that occurs concomitant with cardiac disease.

Foetal distress occurs early in labour if the foetal condition is already impaired. However, it may occur later if there have been untoward events during the process of labour, such as retroplacental bleeding, compression or entanglement of the umbilical cord, hypotension caused by epidural anaesthesia, or prolonged labour for any reason. In brief, the causes of foetal distress can be thought of as falling into several categories, namely maternal, uterine, placental and foetal – to which must be added a number of problems involving the umbilical cord. The outcome of foetal distress is very variable as infants are, on the whole, surprisingly resilient with only 1% of infants being severely asphyxiated at birth (Apgar score of 0–3 at 5 min) suffering subsequent cerebral palsy. However, there are a number of features that can provide useful information in assessing the prognosis as regards development of postanoxic encephalopathy. These include level of consciousness, degree of neuromuscular control, establishment of complex reflexes, autonomic function, electroencephalography and duration of clinical disturbance[155,156]. The main cause of postnatal hypoxia is the respiratory distress syndrome (RDS), in which deficiency of pulmonary surfactant has caused formation of hyaline membranes; the latter line the alveolar ducts, alveoli and respiratory bronchioles of those infants who survive the first eight hours of life. In consequence there is hypoxia, hypercapnia and mixed respiratory and metabolic acidosis. In the case of cyanotic congenital heart disease, although there may be marked hypoxaemia, there is often adequate oxygen saturation for the needs of tissue respiration; hence, severe acidosis does not necessarily occur.

Biochemical basis[155,156]

In newborn infants metabolism is biased towards the anaerobic or glycolytic pathway and on this account there is greater relative tolerance to episodes of hypoxia than at any other time of life. Nevertheless, should oxygenation not be established quickly then glycogen reserves are soon exhausted and acidosis, both metabolic and respiratory, will ensue both rapidly and progressively; the infant will exhibit cyanosis and apnoea. However, the major consideration must be that the outcome of depressed cerebral function in such an infant may well lead to permanent brain injury. Should hypoxia continue to increase then the infant will display pallor and apnoea and death will ensue. Severe intrapartum hypoxia is often followed by moderate renal failure and there is sometimes hyperammonaemia, consequent on hepatic ischaemia. It has also been reported that metabolites of hypoxanthine are found in the CSF after intrapartum asphyxia.

Hyperbilirubinaemia[157,158]

Clinical aspects

Neonatal jaundice becomes clinically recognizable when the serum bilirubin level exceeds a value of 85 μmol/l; the jaundice in the majority of these is regarded as physiological. There are a number of pathological disorders, however, which can themselves cause a further rise of bilirubin over and above the level seen physiologically. Some of the more important of these disorders are haemolysis, increased red cell mass, infections, dehydration, insufficient energy intake, hypoxia, hypothyroidism, hypoglycaemia and galactosaemia. Furthermore, prematurity, poorly controlled maternal diabetes mellitus, the presence of Down syndrome and the prolonged jaundice sometimes associated with breast feeding can all be responsible for adding to the bilirubin load. Unconjugated bilirubin is a toxic substance if present in excess and can, in the neonate, produce either a transient encephalopathy or irreversible damage to the brain. Classic kernicterus does not usually occur unless the serum bilirubin exceeds 340 μmol/l, although values of 205–340 μmol/l do seem to be associated with an increased incidence of neurodevelopmental delay during the first year of life. Indications that there is a toxic level of unconjugated bilirubin in the neonate include the presence of irritability or lethargy, poor sucking and the development of an abnormal brain-stem auditory evoked response[159]; further neurological signs appear as kernicterus develops, including opisthotonus, seizures and a high-pitched cry. These presentations eventually diminish, assuming the neonate survives, but are replaced by overt extrapyramidal signs and the appearance of mental retardation. There are many factors influencing the relationship between blood levels of unconjugated bilirubin and the onset of brain damage. Some may escape such damage at high levels, whereas others may be unfortunate enough to express bilirubin encephalopathy or deafness at relatively low levels.

Biochemical basis

Death at the height of kernicterus is associated with intense yellow staining of many of the cortical nuclei of the brain; the neurones show swelling, the cytoplasm becomes increasingly granular and cell inclusions due to bilirubin–membrane complexes may appear. Bilirubin is toxic on account of its ability to damage membranes; in consequence there can be leakage of ions, inhibition of electron transport, inhibition of synthesis of DNA and protein and uncoupling of oxidative phosporylation.

Iron deficiency[160]

Clinical aspects

Many research studies have revealed that in children poor levels of development and cognitive function occur in the presence of iron deficiency; behavioural differences have also been noted. Nevertheless, it is not always possible to draw accurate conclusions from such studies on account of the poor social circumstances in which many of the individuals lived. This could itself be contributory to the clinical situation, perhaps causing confusion in interpretation of the findings for many reasons. Nevertheless, there does seem to be strong evidence in developing countries that, in the presence of iron deficiency anaemia, children are likely to gain benefit, in the form of improved cognitive function and school achievement, from receiving iron treatment. It has been convincingly demonstrated that dietary ferrous sulfate, given for a period of 4 months to infants of 12–18 months of age suffering from iron deficiency, resulted in raising mental and motor development levels to those of infants where there was sufficiency of iron[161].

Biochemical basis

There has been a problem in accurately defining what is meant by iron deficiency but on the whole it is accepted that from analysis of blood at least two iron indices should be found to be abnormal before it is considered established. The evidence is that it takes a considerable time for significant improvement to be seen in developmental attainment of the child in response to iron treatment. This would be consistent with the better responses observed in long-term research studies when compared with those of shorter duration. It may well be important to keep in mind the long time lapse from instituting iron therapy to attainment of a satisfactory response, when attempting to identify the precise underlying biochemical mechanisms involved.

Protein-energy malnutrition (PEM)[160,162]

Clinical aspects

Protein-energy malnutrition (PEM), in its various forms, is estimated to be present in 100 million children throughout the world. It has traditionally been regarded as a spectrum of disorders ranging from marasmus to kwashiorkor. Of special interest is the observation that the effects of such malnutrition can be, at least partially, overcome by certain environmental stimuli. In one study, for instance, there was opportunity to observe malnourished Korean girls following placement at an early stage into middle class American families. They were examined after 6 years and were found to have IQ and achievement scores which surpassed not only those of the average Korean child of the same age but also those of the average American child. Nevertheless, children who were more severely malnourished, but treated in the same way, were still found to lag behind the two control groups when followed at a later stage[163]. Furthermore, there is recognition that the spectrum of PEM is even more widely spread than this; there may be degrees of PEM, albeit not as severe as is seen in marasmus or kwashiorkor, in every hospital paediatric ward; moreover, such presentations may well be of relatively short duration and, therefore, merely temporary. The nutritional deficiencies, in these instances, are secondary to the diseases from which the children are suffering or, perhaps it is consequent upon the family and social circumstances into which the infant has been born.

Severely malnourished children in the acute stage of severe PEM display apathy and inactivity and tend to be more reluctant to explore. However, following institution of proper dietary management there is rapid recovery towards normal. Information on the long-term effects of severe PEM has come largely from studying school-aged children who, in the earlier part of their lives, had experienced severe malnutrition. The evidence from several such studies seems to be that the children had a lower IQ when they were assessed several years later and that this lower level persisted; in addition, there were also seen to be accompanying behaviour problems, poorer school achievement, a poor performance in memory tests and delay in motor development[160].

Marasmus[164] is characterized by initial failure to gain weight and is followed by actual loss of weight on account of muscle wasting and depletion of sub-cutaneous fat; eventually there is emaciation (weight can fall to as much as 30% of that expected in relation to age of the infant). Although at first it is not common for there to be loss of appetite it does subsequently diminish. The lack of oedema in marasmus is in marked contrast to the presence of marked oedema in kwashiorkor, where weight loss is less on account of retention of water which is itself relatively heavy (1.0 litre weighs 1.0 kg). The mood is initially fretful but later the infant becomes listless. Several important causes include failure of lactation, low birth weight and repeated gastrointestinal or other infections; to these can be added various congenital malformations and metabolic abnormalities, together with improper feeding habits perhaps due to a disturbed relationship between parent and child.

Kwashiorkor[164] may be seen any time in the first 5 years of life after weaning has occurred. There is poor appetite, growth retardation and oedema (often coinciding with the presence of a fatty liver). As already noted above, oedema is the feature which distinguishes this condition from marasmus and accounts for the relative lack of weight loss, largely because of the weight of water retained. There is also accompanying disturbance in cellular immunity and gastroenteritis is common. There is a change of mood, too, in the form of general irritability, apathy and listlessness; indeed, the mental effects are more noticeable than in the case of marasmus. In particular, it is regarded as a very good sign when the child regains its ability to smile in response to therapy (i.e. medications, dietary management and sensory stimulation). It is helpful to include sensory stimulation in the formula of rehabilitation of these children as it does seem to play a vital role in aiding a satisfactory outcome.

Biochemical basis

Analyses of the brains of children dying of PEM, whether of marasmic or kwashiorkor type, show that there are fewer cells (as indicated by a lower DNA content) (Figure 19)[113] and less myelin than in the brains of normal children of the same age; nevertheless, the amounts of DNA present seem to be appropriate for the actual brain weight (Figure 20)[113]. In contrast, measurements of dendritic/synaptic growth using a specific ganglioside (the disialoganglioside, G_{D1a}) as marker, show that dendritic growth appears to be specifically reduced by malnutrition (Figure 21)[113]. Other work, however, has indicated that sensory stimulation induces dendritic growth. We may, therefore, conclude that sensory deprivation may contribute substantially to the manifestations of poor dendritic arborization in the brains of malnourished children.

Protein-energy malnutrition (PEM) and its relationship to mental development has been the topic of a number of recent studies. These have concluded that severe PEM equates with kwashiorkor, marasmus and marasmic-kwashiorkor whereas the term 'moderate malnutrition' has been used when weight attainment has been less than 80% of that expected for age and sex. The precise biochemical mechanisms underlying the transient behavioural changes of severe malnutrition and their improvement in response to proper dietary management, was regarded in these studies as being generally unknown.

Marasmus is the result of taking too little of an otherwise reasonably balanced diet; in consequence there is nutritional deficiency of all the normal food components. In severe undernutrition there is no physiological function of the body which does not undergo some degree of reductive adaptation, e.g. metabolic rate, sodium pump activity, protein synthesis, protein breakdown, cardiac output, etc., all show reduced levels of activity during the malnutrition phase.

Kwashiorkor commences in a different way from marasmus; there have been, over the years, many attempts at explaining its development and one such attempt, the protein deficiency theory, is briefly quoted below. It must be said here that most of these hypotheses, including that of protein deficiency, do not adequately account either for the clinical features of the condition as a whole or for its epidemiology. The protein deficiency theory is based on comparison with the nutrition of normal children, in whom consumption of nitrogenous

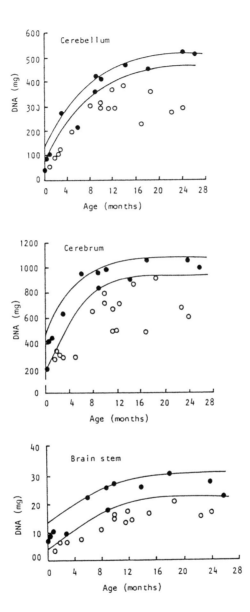

Figure 19 Amount of DNA (indicative of cell numbers) in various parts of the brain of malnourished (○) and control (●) infants (with permission of Dr. Wiruck)

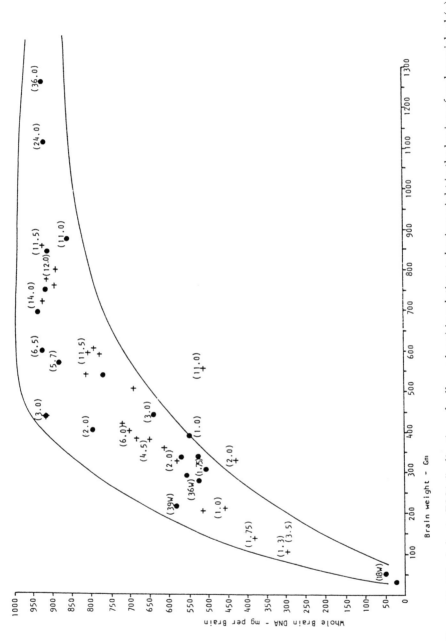

Figure 20 Whole brain DNA (indicative of cell numbers) in relation to brain weight in the brains of malnourished (+) and control (●) infants. The age of the infants (in brackets) is shown prenatally in weeks (w) and postnatally in months

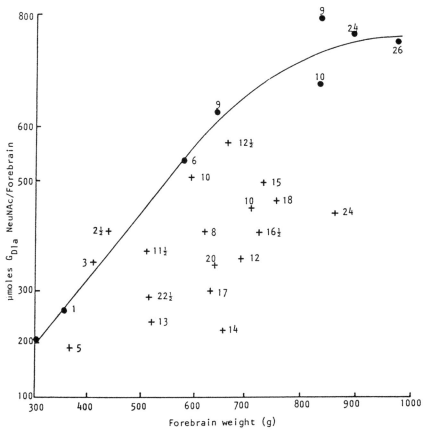

Figure 21 The effect of protein-energy malnutrition (PEM) on the amount of disialoganglioside (G_{D1a}) in the human forebrain. Values for malnourished children (+), control children (•), age in months (with permission of Prof. Dickerson)

food is sufficient to maintain positive nitrogen balance, thereby supplying the needs of growth. The maternal source of high-class animal protein ceases at the time of weaning; hence, other foods, which in developing countries may not be of comparable nutritional value, have to suffice. The theory states that as a result a state of relative protein deficiency develops at this time, which itself causes anorexia; this in turn leads to growing inability to ingest sufficient weaning food with the result that there is deficient energy intake. In support of all this, flattening of the growth curve is usually seen at this time. An alternative theory, however, has now been advanced which attributes clinical presentation of the patient to imbalance between production of free radicals and the safe disposal thereof[162]. The important consequence of this idea is that marasmus and kwashiorkor are no longer the two ends of a spectrum with marasmus representing pure energy deficiency and kwashiorkor equating with pure protein deficiency, and all the intermediate states being regarded as various grades of protein-energy malnutrition, but that these two disorders are aetiologically separate. Marasmus, therefore, would be caused by a combination of energy and protein deficiency, whereas kwashiorkor would be secondary to various stresses and provocations (e.g. infections and toxins) being superimposed upon a patient whose antioxidant and free radical protective mechanisms were compromised[162]. A diet that is lacking in the components, needed to maintain adequate free radical protection (e.g. sulfur-containing amino acids, zinc, copper and manganese), is often concomitantly deficient in energy and protein content also. Marasmus and kwashiorkor can, therefore, coexist in the same population, although there are some populations where marasmus is common and kwashiorkor rare and *vice versa*. It is essential to realise that the many conditions which can act as precipitants of kwashiorkor also concomitantly provoke increased free radical flux at the same time; the result is that there is lessened available protection from these normally protective pathways. A large number of recognised nutrients (including vitamin E, vitamin A, carotene, sulfur-containing amino acids, copper, zinc, manganese, iron, selenium, riboflavin, nicotinic acid, magnesium and thiamine) are now clearly involved in this protective scheme; a lessened intake of even a portion of these could surely impair the ability of the body to tolerate radical producing stresses[162].

Lead poisoning[165,166]

Clinical aspects[166]

It is only in the last 30 years that lead poisoning has come to the fore in being considered a serious public health problem in children. However, controversy still prevails over the long-term effects of lead and indeed, also over the actual level in the blood that equates with what can be regarded as an increased body burden. Several studies have suggested that raised levels are associated with minor neurological dysfunction, including motor coordination problems and difficulties with fine motor control. Moreover, psychological assessment has revealed low-average mental ability, deficiency in adaptive behaviour, deficit in language function, reduced IQ and hyperactive behaviour but, on the other hand, some research investigations have revealed no differences between test and control subjects.

At a higher level of lead intake (i.e. blood lead level of greater than 2.0 μmol/l) the early symptoms of lead poisoning comprise anorexia, irritability, drowsiness and apathy. In addition, the child may exhibit lessened interest in playing activities and there may be episodes of abdominal pain. Following even greater intake there is a more serious expression of lead toxicity in the form of vomiting, apathy, stupor and ataxia, merging into lead encephalopathy (i.e. blood lead level of greater than 4.0 μmol/l). There is a high mortality with this condition (up to 30%); moreover, 25% of the survivors are left with a deficit of brain function[167]. One study revealed that 5 years after such an episode of lead intoxication the sequelae included an average IQ of only 80, behavioural problems and neurological deficits of several kinds[168].

Biochemical basis

Lead is toxic mainly on account of its effects on the CNS, the peripheral nervous system, the red cells in the bone marrow and the kidney. Lead is an inhibitor of a number of the enzymes involved in incorporating iron into haem – not surprisingly anaemia results. There is also a rise in red cell protoporphyrin. It is the developing nervous system in foetal life and in young children that is particularly sensitive to the presence of this heavy metal. In lead encephalopathy an increase in vascular permeability causes massive cerebral oedema; there is also destruction of neurones. In animal studies it has been found that doses of lead, insufficient in themselves to cause histopathologic changes, can lead to slower learning ability and changes in behaviour[165].

ROLE OF INFANT FEEDING ON COGNITIVE FUNCTION LATER IN LIFE

We have seen that brain maturation and the intelligence subsequently attained are both affected by many determinants, including the complex interplay of nutritional, hormonal, economic and socio-cultural factors. Within this context, the particular relationship between the way in which a newborn baby is fed and the intelligence that finally emerges is a matter, not only of great interest but also of considerable importance. As long ago as 1929[169] it was suggested that breast-fed babies were destined to be advantaged in terms of subsequent IQ. Hence, if breast milk actually provides important constituents for development of the brain, it would be entirely reasonable to expect to see a greater effect from the breast-feeding of premature babies – when the brain grows and develops at a more rapid rate than in those babies born at term. Children born before term who had been given mother's milk were found to have a higher IQ at 7.5–8.0 years of age than those who did not receive mother's milk[170]. Moreover, this difference was found to remain after adjustment for differences in maternal education and social class.

It was considered possible, therefore, that the developmental advantage associated with the feeding of mother's milk might be related to the presence of long-chain polyunsaturated fatty acids (e.g. docosahexanoic acid, DHA) which are known to accumulate in the developing brain and retina; DHA was not present in formula-milks. A retrospective study of full-term infants in Holland, all examined at 9 years of age, indicated that breast-feeding imparted neurological advantage which was also considered by the authors to be possibly attributable to the presence of long-chain polyunsaturated fatty acids in breast milk. Moreover, the essential role of DHA for neural maturation appears to have been confirmed in full-term infants by way of a placebo-controlled study in which formula-feed, supplemented with fish oil (a source of DHA), was found to promote higher visual evoked potential (VEP) acuity compared with the same formula-feed without the added DHA[171].

It is, clearly, essential in any such study, in which there has been attempt to precisely ascertain the effect of infant nutrition, to take into account all the other factors affecting brain function and then to appropriately adjust for them. Among such factors, both social class and maternal education have been considered important but it has been questioned whether they do actually equate with maternal intelligence which is itself known to be related to the intelligence of the offspring[170,172]. Irrespective of social class and education, the fact is that more intelligent women have more intelligent children, no matter how they were fed as babies; in addition, more intelligent women tend to breast feed their babies. In a study of men and women born in Hertfordshire (England) between 1920 and 1930 it was shown that the mechanisms linking the type of feeding in early life to later intelligence were influenced more by social environment than the nutritional qualities of the milk on which they were fed[173]. To conclude this controversial topic relating breast feeding, quality of maternal care of the infant and subsequent intelligence quotient, it does currently seem that intelligent, loving and caring mothers are likely to have intelligent children, irrespective of how they choose to feed their babies[172].

11
Conclusions

The foregoing account of the biochemical and mental aspects of psychiatric disorders has covered some of the more florid conditions (e.g. schizophrenia, depression, mania/hypomania, anxiety and Alzheimer's disease). In addition to the mood changes and psychiatric consequences of biochemical derangements, there has been reference to pharmacological, toxicological and nutritional causes too. Furthermore, a feature of the text has been a chapter on the psychiatric consequences of disorders of the developing brain.

It is clear that O_2 and glucose are so fundamental a requirement for cerebral processes that sudden depletion of either will rapidly terminate consciousness. However, assuming there is sufficient oxygen and glucose present, then there is still a vast array of other mechanisms which, should they falter, could distort the finely tuned biochemical and physiological architecture of the mind. Hence, there would be created disturbances of mood, memory and intellect. The final outcome of disorders of neurotransmitters, neuromodulators, neurohormones and neuromediators is the basis of much of the general practice of psychiatry. Furthermore, encephalopathic processes secondary to deviations of metabolism may be due to the presence of too much metabolite (e.g. renal failure, etc.) or too little of an essential component (e.g. the pyrophosphate derivative of vitamin B_1 which serves as coenzyme in many enzymic reactions, etc.), thus moulding behaviour, thoughts and feelings in yet different ways. Even too much water (e.g. SIADH), with its consequential dilutional effect on the electrolytes at neuronal membrane level, will slow and depress mental processes, as also does (but via a very different mechanism) depletion of that overall determinant of the rate of metabolic processes – thyroxine. Other endocrine hormones exert their own specific influences in different ways. Moreover, all these factors – and others – may have different consequences at varying stages in the life-cycle of the individual.

It should be reiterated that the disorders discussed so far have been, essentially, biochemically induced or based. The mental accompaniments of physical lesions (e.g. the depression associated with space-occupying lesions of the brain, etc.) and of those disorders of microbiological origin (e.g. the fatigue that may precede or accompany viral hepatitis and which may, in subclinical cases, be the only symptom; the dementia of HIV infection, etc.) have been specifically excluded; nevertheless, all of them need to be considered during the process of differential diagnosis.

Finally, it seems appropriate to return to J.W.L. Thudichum and to the prophetic words he wrote in 1884, surely as true today as when they were written[174]. On the final pages of his great treatise on the chemical constituents of the brain he writes, 'I believe that the great diseases of the brain and spine, such as general paralysis, acute and chronic mania, melancholy, and others, will all be shown to be connected with specific chemical changes in neuroplasm, the products of which cannot be more complicated than the chemolytic products of the educts; they need, however, not be identical with chemolytic products, but may be new morbid products. Here is a field for inquiry of the possession of which the guardians of refuges for the insane will hereafter, I have no doubt, endeavour to make good use'[174]. He ends the volume by saying, 'In short, it is probable that by the aid of chemistry many derangements of the brain and mind, which are at present obscure, will become accurately definable and amenable to precise treatment, and what is now an object of anxious empiricism will become one for the proud exercise of exact science'[174].

Abbreviations

ACh	acetylcholine
AChE	acetylcholinesterase
ACTH	adrenocorticotrophic hormone
ADH	antidiuretic hormone
AII	angiotensin II
AIP	acute intermittent porphyria
δ-ALA	δ-aminolevulinic acid
ALT	alanine transaminase
ALTE	acute life-threatening episodes
ANA	antinuclear antibodies
AP	action potential
AP	alkaline phosphatase
AR	aldehyde reductase
AST	aspartate transaminase
ATP	adenosine triphosphate
AVP	arginine vasopressin
cAMP	cyclic adenosine 3′,5′-monophosphate
CAT	choline acetyltransferase
CCK	cholecystokinin
cGMP	cyclic guanosine 3′,5′-monophosphate
CLIP	corticotrophin-like intermediate lobe peptide
CNS	central nervous system
CO	carbon monoxide
CO_2	carbon dioxide
CoA	coenzyme A
COMT	catechol-O-methyltransferase
CRF	corticotrophin releasing factor
CSF	cerebrospinal fluid
CT	computerized tomography
DA	dopamine
DBH	dopamine β-hydroxylase
δ-ALA	delta-aminolevulinic acid
DET	diethyltryptamine

DHA	docosahexanoic acid
DMT	dimethyltryptamine
DNA	deoxyribonucleic acid
DOM	2,5-dimethoxy-4-methyl-amphetamine
DOPA	dihydroxyphenylalanine
DOPAC	dihydroxyphenylacetic acid
DOPEG	3,4-dihydroxyphenylethylene glycol
DOPGAL	3,4-dihydroxyphenylglycoaldehyde
DST	dexamethasone suppression test
ECF	extracellular fluid
ECG	electrocardiogram
ECT	electroconvulsive therapy
EEG	electroencephalogram
ESR	erythrocyte sedimentation rate
FBC	full blood count
FSH	follicle-stimulating hormone
FT_4	free thyroxine
GABA	gamma-aminobutyric acid
GABA-T	gamma-aminobutyric acid transaminase
GAD	glutamic acid decarboxylase
GH	growth hormone
GTT	glucose tolerance test
5HIAA	5-hydroxyindoleacetic acid
H_2O	water
5HT	serotonin
5HTP	5-hydroxytryptophan
HVA	homovanillic acid
IDDM	insulin-dependent diabetes mellitus
IQ	intelligence quotient
IUGR	intrauterine growth retardation
K^+	potassium
KAI	kainic acid
LDH	lactate dehydrogenase
LH	luteinizing hormone
LNAA	large neutral amino acids
LPH	lipotrophin
LSD	lysergic acid diethylamide
MAO	monoamine oxidase

MAOI	monoamine oxidase inhibitor
MCV	mean corpuscular volume
MEN	multiple endocrine neoplasia
MEOS	microsomal ethanol oxidizing system
MOPEG	3-methoxy-4-hydroxyphenylethylene glycol
MSH	melanocyte stimulating hormone
MSUD	maple syrup urine disease
NA	noradrenaline
Na^+	sodium
NAD	nicotinamide adenine dinucleotide (oxidized)
NADH	nicotinamide adenine dinucleotide (reduced)
NADP	nicotinamide adenine dinucleotide phosphate (oxidized)
NADPH	nicotinamide adenine dinucleotide phosphate (reduced)
NGF	nerve growth factor
NH_3	ammonia
NH_4^+	ammonium
NIDDM	non-insulin dependent diabetes mellitus
NMDA	*N*-methyl-D-aspartate
NT	neurotensin
OAF	osteoclast-activating factor
PBG	porphobilinogen
PC	phosphate clearance
PCO_2	partial pressure of CO_2
PCP	phencyclidine
PEI	phosphate excretion index
PEM	protein-energy malnutrition
PER	phosphate excretion ratio
PET	positron emission tomography
PKU	phenylketonuria
PNMT	phenylethanolamine *N*-methyltransferase
PO_2	partial pressure of O_2
POMC	pro-opiomelanocortin
PRL	prolactin
PTH	parathyroid hormone
QUIS	quisqualic acid
RA	rheumatoid arthritis
RAS	reticular activating system
RDS	respiratory distress syndrome

REM	rapid eye movement
RNA	ribonucleic acid
RR	reference range
SAD	seasonal affective disorder
SD	standard deviation
SFD	small-for-dates
SG	specific gravity
SGA	small for gestational age
SIADH	syndrome of inappropriate ADH
SNRI	serotonin noradrenaline re-uptake inhibitor
SSRI	selective serotonin re-uptake inhibitor
T_3	tri-iodothyronine
T_4	thyroxine
TCA	tricyclic antidepressant
TDM	therapeutic drug monitoring
THC	tetrahydrocannabinol
TPN	total parenteral nutrition
TPP	thiamine pyrophosphate
TRH	thyrotrophin-releasing hormone
TRP	tubular reabsorption of phosphate
TSH	thyroid-stimulating hormone
VEP	visual evoked potential
VIP	vasoactive intestinal peptide
VMA	vanillylmandelic acid

References

1. Thudichum, J.L.W. (1884). Preface In *A Treatise on the Chemical Constitution of the Brain*, pp. vii–xiii. (London: Baillière, Tindall, and Cox)
2. Kety, S.S. (1959). Biochemical theories of schizophrenia. *Science*, **129**, 1528–32
3. Young, J.Z. (1979). Learning as a process of selection and amplification. *J. R. Soc. Med.*, **72**, 801–14
4. Iversen, L.L. (1979). The chemistry of the brain. *Sci. Am.*, **241**:3, 118–29
5. Donaldson, D. (1984). Causes and mechanisms of hypoglycaemia. *Faculty News (NW London Faculty of the Roy. Coll. Gen. Pract.*, **4**, No. 1, 5–6
6. Bloom, F.E. (1996). Neurotransmission and the central nervous system. In Hardman, J.G., Limbird, L.E., Molinoff, P.B., Ruddon, R.W. and Gilman, A.G. (eds.) *Goodman and Gilman's The Pharmacological Basis of Therapeutics*, 9th edn., pp. 267–93. (New York, London, Tokyo: McGraw-Hill Health Professions Division)
7. McAllister-Williams, R.H. and Young, A.H. (1990). Neuroscience and psychiatry: the decade of the brain. *Psychiatry in Practice*, **9**:3, 12–16
8. Rang, H.P., Dale, M.M., Ritter, J.M. and Gardner, P. (1995). Chemical transmission and drug action in the central nervous system. In *Pharmacology*, pp. 491–518. (New York, London, Melbourne: Churchill Livingstone)
9. Rang, H.P., Dale, M.M., Ritter, J.M. and Gardner, P. (1995). Chemical transmission and the autonomic nervous system. In *Pharmacology*, pp. 101–116. (New York, London, Melbourne: Churchill Livingstone)
10. Hoffman, B.B., Lefkowitz, R.J. and Taylor, P. (1996). Neurotransmission: the autonomic and somatic motor nervous systems. In Hardman, J.G., Limbird, L.E., Molinoff, P.B., Ruddon, R.W. and Gilman, A.G. (eds) *Goodman and Gilman's The Pharmacological Basis of Therapeutics*, 9th edn., pp. 105–39. (New York: McGraw-Hill Health Professions Division)
11. Rang, H.P., Dale, M.M., Ritter, J.M. and Gardner, P. (1995). Noradrenergic transmission. In *Pharmacology*, pp. 148–76. (New York, London, Melbourne: Churchill Livingstone)
12. Ferrier, I.N. (1991). Serotonin in psychiatry. *Br. J. Hosp. Med.*, **45**, 191
13. Bender, D.A. (1978). Regulation of 5-hydroxytryptamine synthesis. *Proc. Nutr. Soc.*, **37**, 159–65

14. Anderson, I.M., Parry-Billings, M., Newsholme, E.A., Fairburn, C.G. and Cowen, P.J. (1990). Dieting reduces plasma tryptophan and alters brain 5-HT function in women. *Psychol. Med.*, **20**, 785–91

15. Rang, H.P., Dale, M.M., Ritter, J.M. and Gardner, P. (1995). Cholinergic transmission. In *Pharmacology*, pp. 117–47. (New York, London, Edinburgh: Churchill Livingstone)

16. Reisine, T. and Pasternak, G. (1996). Opioid analgesics and antagonists. In Hardman, J.G., Limbird, L.E., Molinoff, P.B., Ruddon, R.W. and Gilman, A.G. (eds.) *Goodman and Gilman's The Pharmacological Basis of Therapeutics*, 9th edn., pp. 521–55. (New York, London, Tokyo: McGraw-Hill Health Professions Division)

17. Deakin, W. (1987). Biological mechanisms in the major psychiatric syndromes. *Med. Int.*, **43**, 1764–9

18. Rossor, M. (1993). Disorders of higher cerebral cortical function and behavioural neurology. In Walton J. (ed.) *Brain's Diseases of the Nervous System*, 10th edn., pp. 740–67. (Oxford, New York, Tokyo: Oxford University Press)

19. Guyton, A.C. and Hall, J.E. (1996). The cerebral cortex; intellectual functions of the brain; and learning and memory. In *Textbook of Medical Physiology*, 9th edn., pp. 733–47. (Philadelphia, London, Montreal: W.B. Saunders Co.)

20. Growden, J.H. and Young, R.H. (1994). Paralysis and movement disorders. In Isselbacher, K.J., Braunwald, E., Wilson, J.D., Martin, J.B., Fauci, A.S. and Kasper, D.L. (eds.) *Harrison's Principles of Internal Medicine*, 13th edn., pp. 115–25. (New York, London, Toronto: McGraw-Hill Inc.)

21. Guyton, A.C. (1992). Activation of the brain; wakefulness and sleep; behavioural functions of the brain. In *Human Physiology and Mechanisms of Disease*, 7th edn., pp. 447–58. (Philadelphia, London, Toronto: W.B. Saunders Co.)

22. Guyton, A.C. and Hall, J.E. (1996). Behavioural and motivational mechanisms of the brain – the limbic system and hypothalamus. In *Textbook of Medical Physiology*, 9th edn., pp. 749–60. (Philadelphia, London, Montreal: W.B. Saunders Co.)

23. Berry, M.M., Bannister, L.H. and Standring, S.M. (1995). The limbic lobe and olfactory pathways. In Bannister, L.H., Berry, M.M., Collins, P., Dyson, M., Dussek, J.E. and Ferguson, M.W.J. (eds.) *Gray's Anatomy*, 38th edn., pp. 1115–41. (New York, London, Melbourne: Churchill Livingstone)

24. Walton, J. (1993). Disorders of the autonomic nervous system and hypothalamus. In Walton, J. (ed.) *Brain's Diseases of the Nervous System*,

10th edn., pp. 677–89. (Oxford, New York, Tokyo: Oxford University Press)

25. Hall, R. (1987). Pituitary and hypothalamic disorders. In Weatherall, D.J., Ledingham, J.G.G. and Warrell, D.A. (eds.) *Oxford Textbook of Medicine*, 2nd edn, Volume 1, pp. 10.7–10.30. (Oxford, Melbourne, New York: Oxford University Press)

26. Thorner, M.O. (1996). Anterior pituitary disorders. In Weatherall, D.J., Ledingham, J.G.G. and Warrell, D.A. (eds.) *Oxford Textbook of Medicine*, 3rd edn., Volume 2, pp. 1573–99. (Oxford, New York, Tokyo: Oxford University Press)

27. Jameson, J.L. (1996). Principles of hormone action. In Weatherall, D.J., Ledingham, J.G.G. and Warrell, D.A. (eds.) *Oxford Textbook of Medicine*, 3rd edn., Volume 2, pp. 1553–73. (Oxford, New York, Tokyo: Oxford University Press)

28. Guyton, A.C. and Hall, J.E. (1996). States of brain activity – sleep; brain waves; epilepsy; psychoses. In *Textbook of Medical Physiology*, 9th edn., pp. 761–8. (Philadelphia, London, Montreal: W.B. Saunders Co.)

29. Ropper, A.H. and Martin, J.B. (1994). Coma and other disorders of consciousness. In Isselbacher, K.J., Braunwald, E., Wilson, J.D., Martin, J.B., Fauci, A.S. and Kasper, D.L. (eds.) *Harrison's Principles of Internal Medicine*, 13th edn., pp. 146–53. (New York, London, Madrid: McGraw-Hill Inc.)

30. Perry, E.K. (1991). Neurotransmitters and diseases of the brain. *Br. J. Hosp. Med.*, **45**, 73–83

31. Beal, M.F., Richardson, E.P. Jr. and Martin, J.B. (1994). Alzheimer's disease and other dementias. In Isselbacher, K.J., Braunwald, E., Wilson, J.D., Martin, J.B., Fauci, A.S. and Kasper, D.L. (eds.) *Harrison's Principles of Internal Medicine*, 13th edn., pp. 2269–75. (New York, New Delhi, Toronto: McGraw-Hill Inc.)

32. Kistler, J.P., Ropner, A.H. and Martin, J.B. (1994). Cerebrovascular diseases. In Isselbacher, K.J., Braunwald, E., Wilson, J.D., Martin, J.B., Fauci, A.S. and Kasper, D.L. (eds.) *Harrison's Principles of Internal Medicine*, 13th edn., pp. 2233–56. (New York, London, Sydney: McGraw-Hill Inc.)

33. Valenstein, E. and Heilman, K.M. (1979). Emotional disorders resulting from lesions of the central nervous system. In Heilman, K.M. and Valenstein, E. (eds.) *Clinical Neuropsychology*, pp. 413–38. (New York, Oxford: Oxford University Press)

34. Ganong, W.F. (1995). Neural basis of instinctual behavior and emotions. In *Review of Medical Physiology*, 17th edn., pp. 233–42. (London, Sydney, Toronto: Prentice-Hall International Inc)

35. Electricwala, A., Donaldson, D., Vaddadi, K.S. and Sherwood, R.F. (1986). Schizophrenia: biochemical theories. *Psychiatry in Practice*, February, 12–13

36. Cooper, J.E. (1991). Schizophrenia and allied conditions. *Med. Int.*, **94**, 3917–22

37. Yakeley, J.W. and Murray, R.M. (1996). Schizophrenia. *Medicine*, **24**:2, 6–10

38. Laurence, D.R. and Bennett, P.N. (1992). Central nervous system III: Drugs and mental disorder – psychotropic and psychoactive drugs. In *Clinical Pharmacology*, 7th edn., pp. 275–301. (Edinburgh, London, New York: Churchill Livingstone)

39. Thompson, C. (1996). Mood disorders. *Medicine*, **24**:2, 1–5

40. Mander, A.J. and Goodwin, G.M. (1990). Neuroendocrinology of psychiatric disorders. *Hospital Update*, March, 211–27

41. Gelder, M. (1991). Diagnosis and management of anxiety and phobic disorders. *Med. Int.*, **94**, 3913–17

42. Peveler, R. and Baldwin, D. (1996). Anxiety disorders. *Medicine*, **24**:2, 11–14

43. Davison, A. (1985). The pathophysiology of dementia. *Pract. Rev. Psychiatry*. Published by Education in Practice, Medical Tribune Group, sponsored by E.R. Squibb and Sons, No. **6**, 1–4

44. Ring, H. (1996). Dementia and delirium. *Medicine*, **24**:3, 51–4

45. Gottfries, C.G. (1990). Neurochemical changes in the human brain and their importance for behaviour in the senium. *Triangle* (Sandoz Journal of Medical Science), **29**, No. 2/3, 127–31

46. Arendt, J. (1991). Melatonin in humans: jet-lag and after. In Arendt, J. and Pevet, P. (eds.) *Advances in Pineal Research* no. 5, pp. 299–302. (London, Paris, Rome: John Libbey)

47. Donaldson, D. (1981). Biological rhythms and medicine. *Update*, February, 309–14

48. Wurtman, R.J. and Wurtman, J.J. (1989). Carbohydrates and depression. *Sci. Am.*, January, 50–7

49. Kendell, R.E., Chalmers, J.C. and Platz, C. (1987). Epidemiology of puerperal psychosis. *Br. J. Psychiatry*, **150**, 662–73

50. Deakin, J.F.W. (1986). Neuro-endocrine aspects of puerperal psychiatric illness. *Pract. Rev. Psychiatry* (Published by Education in Practice, Medical Tribune Group, sponsored by E.R. Squibb and Sons), No. **9**, 5–8

51. Brockington, I.F. (1987). Menstrual and pregnancy related disorders. *Med. Int.*, **44**, 1811–14

52. Wieck, A., Kumar, R., Hirst, A.D., Marks, M.N., Campbell, I.C. and Checkley, S.A. (1991). Increased sensitivity of dopamine receptors and

recurrence of affective psychosis after childbirth. *Br. Med. J.*, **303**, 613–16

53. Cowen, P.J. Anderson, I.M. and Gartside, S.E. (1990). Endocrinological responses to 5-HT. *Ann. NY Acad. Sci.*, **600**, 250–9

54. Lascelles, P.T. and Donaldson, D. (1989). Dexamethasone suppression test (DST) – single low dose for depression. In *Diagnostic Function Tests in Chemical Pathology*, pp. 43–4. (Dordrecht, Boston, London: Kluwer Academic Publishers)

55. Trimble, M.R. (1996). Affective disorders. In *Biological Psychiatry*, 2nd edn., pp. 226–65. (Chichester, New York: John Wiley and Sons)

56. Lascelles, P.T. and Donaldson, D. (1989). Thyrotrophin-releasing hormone (TRH) stimulation test – intravenous procedure. In *Diagnostic Function Tests in Chemical Pathology*, pp. 144–6. (Dordrecht, Boston, London: Kluwer Academic Publishers)

57. Lascelles, P.T. and Donaldson, D. (1989). Clonidine stimulation test. In *Diagnostic Function Tests in Chemical Pathology*, pp. 29–30. (Dordrecht, Boston, London: Kluwer Academic Publishers)

58. Steptoe, A. (1990). Psychobiological stress responses. In Johnston, M. and Wallace, L. (eds.) *Stress and Medical Procedures*, pp. 3–24. (Oxford, New York, Tokyo: Oxford University Press)

59. Deahl, M.P. (1996). Post-traumatic stress disorder. *Medicine*, **24**:2, 15–16

60. Judd, L.L., Britton, K.T. and Broff, D.L. (1994). Mental disorders. In Isselbacher, K.J., Braunwald, E., Wilson, J.D., Martin, J.B., Fauci, A.S. and Kasper, D.L. (eds.) *Harrison's Principles of Internal Medicine*, 13th edn., pp. 2400–19. (New York, London,Tokyo: McGraw-Hill Inc.)

61. Donaldson, D. (1994). Psychiatric disorders of biochemical origin. In Williams, D.L. and Marks, V. (eds.) *Scientific Foundations of Biochemistry in Clinical Practice*, 2nd edn., pp. 144–60. (Oxford, Boston, Sydney: Butterworth–Heinemann Medical Books Ltd)

62. Lishman, W.A. (1987). Endocrine diseases and metabolic disorders. In *Organic Psychiatry, The Psychological Consequences of Cerebral Disorder*, 2nd edn., pp. 428–85. (Oxford, London, Melbourne: Blackwell Scientific Publications)

63. Katschnig, H. and Amering, M. (1990). The menopause and psychological disorders. *Triangle (Sandoz J. Med. Sci.)*, **29**, No. 2/3, 107–18

64. Charlton, B.G. and Ferrier, I.N. (1989). Hypothalamo-pituitary-adrenal axis abnormalities in depression: a review and a model. *Psychol. Med.*, **19**, 331–6

65. Fava, G.A., Sonino, N. and Morphy, M.A. (1987). Major depression associated with endocrine disease. *Psychiatric Develop.*, **4**, 321–48

66. Granner, D.K. (1996). Thyroid hormones. In Murray, R.K., Granner, D.K., Mayers, P.A. and Rodwell, V.W. (eds.). *Harper's Biochemistry*, 24th edn., pp. 533–8. (London, Tokyo, New Jersey: Prentice-Hall International Inc.)

67. Szabadi, E. (1991). Thyroid dysfunction and affective illness. *Br. Med. J.*, **302**, 923–4

68. Anon. (1980). I had a phaeochromocytoma. *Lancet*, **1**, 922–3

69. Alberti, K.G.M.M. (1978). Metabolic comas and confusions. *Med. Int.*, **10**, 507–15

70. Bachelard, H.S. (1990). The molecular basis of coma and stroke. In Cohen, R.D., Lewis, B., Alberti, K.G.M.M. and Denman, A.M. (eds.). *The Metabolic and Molecular Basis of Acquired Disease*, pp. 1354–80. (London, Sydney, Tokyo: Baillière Tindall)

71. Victor, M. and Martin, J.B. (1994). Nutritional and metabolic diseases of the nervous system. In Isselbacher, K.J., Braunwald, E., Wilson, J.D., Martin, J.B., Fauci, A.S. and Kasper, D.L. (eds.) *Harrison's Principles of Internal Medicine*, 13th edn., pp. 2328–39. (New York, London, Paris: McGraw-Hill Inc.)

72. Lockwood, W. (1985). A night in October. *Aesculapius* (The University of Birmingham Medical and Dental Graduates Society), June, No. 5, 39

73. Patten, J. (1977). Attacks of altered consciousness. In *Neurological Differential Diagnosis: An Illustrated Approach*. pp. 231–7. (London: Harold Starke Ltd)

74. Lishman, W.A. (1987). Toxic disorders. In *Organic Psychiatry, The Psychological Consequences of Cerebral Disorder*, 2nd edn., pp. 508–44. (Oxford, London, Edinburgh: Blackwell Scientific Publications)

75. Vale, A. (1989). Alcohol intoxication and alcohol withdrawal. *Med. Int.*, **62**, 2543–47

76. Horn, D.B. (1985). Biochemical aspects of alcohol. *Med. Int.*, **15**, 649–51

77. Marks, V. (1983). Clinical pathology of alcohol. *J. Clin. Pathol.*, **36**, 365–78

78. Schuckit, M.A. (1994). Alcohol and alcoholism. In Isselbacher, K.J., Braunwald, E., Wilson, J.D., Martin, J.B., Fauci, A.S. and Kasper, D.L. (eds.) *Harrison's Principles of Internal Medicine*, 13th edn., pp. 2420–5. (New York, Sydney, Tokyo: McGraw-Hill Inc.)

79. Rosalki, S.B. (1994). The clinical biochemistry of alcohol. In Williams, D.L. and Marks, V. (eds.) *Scientific Foundations of Biochemistry in Clinical Practice*, 2nd edn., pp. 121–43. (Oxford, Munich, Sydney: Butterworth–Heinemann Medical Books Ltd)

80. Howells, R.B. (1997). Toxic, metabolic and endocrine disorders. In Stein, G. and Wilkinson, G. (eds.) *Seminars in General Adult Psychiatry*, pp. 1103–75. (London: Gaskell)

81. Cumming, A.D. and Swainson, C.P. (1995). Disturbances in water, electrolyte and acid–base balance. In Edwards, C.R.W., Bouchier, I.A.D., Haslett, C. and Chilvers, E.R. (eds.) *Davidson's Principles and Practice of Medicine*, 17th edn., pp. 585–609. (Edinburgh, Melbourne, New York: Churchill Livingstone)

82. Lascelles, P.T. and Lewis, P.D. (1972). Hypodipsia and hypernatraemia associated with hypothalamic and suprasellar lesions. *Brain*, **95**, 249–64

83. McGouran, R.C.M. (1975). Case of salt overdosage. *Br. Med. J.*, **4**, 386

84. Lishman, W.A. (1987). Vitamin deficiencies. In *Organic Psychiatry, The Psychological Consequences of Cerebral Disorder*, 2nd edn., pp. 486–507. (Oxford, London, Edinburgh: Blackwell Scientific Publications)

85. Trimble, M.R., Corbett, J.A. and Donaldson, D. (1980). Folic acid and mental symptoms in children with epilepsy. *J. Neurol. Neurosurg. Psychiatry*, **43**, 1030–4

86. Linter, C.M. (1985). Neuropsychiatric aspects of trace elements. *Br. J. Hosp. Med.*, **34**, 361–5

87. Bridges, K.R. and Bunn, H.F. (1994). Anaemias with disturbed iron metabolism. In Isselbacher, K.J., Braunwald, E., Wilson, J.D., Martin, J.B., Fauci, A.S. and Kasper, D.L. (eds.) *Harrison's Principles of Internal Medicine*, 13th edn., pp. 1721–6. (New York, London, Toronto: McGraw-Hill Inc.)

88. Scrimshaw, N.S. (1991). Iron deficiency. *Sci. Am.*, October, 24–30

89. Graef, J.W. (1994). Heavy metal poisoning. In Isselbacher, K.J., Braunwald, E., Wilson, J.D., Martin, J.B., Fauci, A.S. and Kasper, D.L. (eds.) *Harrison's Principles of Internal Medicine*, 13th edn., pp. 2461–6. (New York, London, Sydney: McGraw-Hill Inc.)

90. Falchuk, K.H. (1994). Disturbances in trace element metabolism. In Isselbacher, K.J., Braunwald, E., Wilson, J.D., Martin, J.B., Fauci, A.S. and Kasper, D.L. (eds.) *Harrison's Principles of Internal Medicine*, 13th edn., pp. 481–3. (New York, London, Sydney: McGraw-Hill Inc.)

91. Stern, J. and Wilcox, A.H. (1994). Inherited and acquired mental deficiency. In Williams, D.L. and Marks, V. (eds.) *Scientific Foundations of Biochemistry in Clinical Practice*, 2nd edn., pp. 253–91. (Oxford, Boston, Sydney: Butterworh–Heinemann Medical Books Ltd)

92. Stern, J. (1985). Biochemical aspects of mental handicap. *Pract. Rev. Psychiatry* (Published by Education in Practice, Medical Tribune Group, sponsored by E.R. Squibb and Sons), No. **2**, 1–3

93. Brennan, M.J.W. and Cantrill, R.C. (1979). Delta-Amino-laevulinic acid is a potent agonist for GABA autoreceptors. *Nature*, **280**, 514–15

94. Ayub, N., Donaldson, D., Bedford, D., Alloway, R. and Ryalls, M. (1997). Hyperactivity and confusion in the presentation of hyoscine overdose. *J. Roy. S. H.*, **117**(4), 242–4

95. Bateman, D.N. (1989). Poisoning with psychotropic drugs. *Med. Int.*, **61**, 2530–4

96. Cowen, P.J. (1991). Drugs and ECT. *Medicine*, 24:2, 17–22

97. O'Brien, C.P. (1988). Drug abuse and dependence. In Wyngaarden, J.B. and Smith, L.H. (eds.) *Cecil Textbook of Medicine*, 18th edn., pp. 52–61. (Philadelphia, London, Tokyo: W.B. Saunders Co.)

98. Vale, J.A. and Meredith, T.J. (1981). Poisonous plants and fungi. In Vale, J.A. and Meredith, T.J. (eds.) *Poisoning – Diagnosis and Treatment*, pp. 193–201. (London, Dordrecht, Boston: Update Books)

99. Hayman, J. (1985). Datura poisoning – the Angel's trumpet. *Pathology*, **17**, 465–6

100. Vale, J.A. and Meredith, T.J. (1981). Poisoning due to marine animals. In Vale, J.A. and Meredith, T.J. (eds.) *Poisoning – Diagnosis and Treatment*, pp. 168–70. (London, Dordrecht, Boston: Update Books)

101. Sakula, A. (1978). Munchausen: fact and fiction. *J. R. Coll. Physicians*, **12**:3, 286–92

102. Hewko, R.A. (1992). Approach to the patient with psychiatric disorders with neurologic symptoms. In Kelley, W.N., DeVita, V.T., DuPont, H.L., Harris, E.D., Hazzard, W.R., Holmes, E.W., Hudson, L.D., Humes, H.D., Paty, D.W., Watanabe, A.M. and Yamada.T. (eds.) *Textbook of Internal Medicine*, 2nd edn., pp. 2294–6. (Philadelphia, New York, London: J.B. Lippincott Co.)

103. Donaldson, D. (1994). Polyuria and disorders of thirst. In Williams, D.L. and Marks, V. (eds.) *Scientific Foundations of Biochemistry in Clinical Practice*, 2nd edn., pp. 76–102. (Oxford, Munich, Sydney: Butterworth–Heinemann Medical Books Ltd)

104. Donaldson, D. (1981). Laboratory investigations in psychiatric disorders. *Faculty News (NW London Faculty of the R. Coll. Gen. Pract.)*, **1**, No. 2, 4

105. Schorah, C.J. and Smithels, R.W. (1991). Maternal vitamin nutrition and malformations of the neural tube. *Nutr. Res. Rev.*, **4**, 33–49

106. Berry, M. (1982). The development of the human nervous system. In Dickerson, J.W.T. and McGurk, H. (eds.) *Brain and Behavioural Development*, pp. 6–47. (Glasgow, London: Surrey University Press (Blackie))

107. Davison, A.N. and Dobbing, J. (1968). The developing brain. In Davison, A.N. and Dobbing, J. (eds.) *Applied Neurochemistry*, pp. 253–86. (Oxford, London, Edinburgh: Blackwell Scientific Publications)

108. Morgan, B.L.G. and Dickerson, J.W.T. (1982). Comparative aspects of brain growth and development. In Dickerson, J.W.T. and McGurk, H. (eds.) *Brain and Behavioural Development*, pp. 48–72. (Glasgow, London: Surrey University Press (Blackie))

109. Dobbing, J. and Sands, J. (1973). The quantitative growth and development of the human brain. *Arch. Dis. Childh.* **48**, 757–67

110. Yakovlev, P. I. and Lecours, A.-R. (1967). The myelogenetic cycles of regional maturation of the brain. In Minkowski, A. (ed.) *Regional Development of the Brain in Early Life*, pp. 3–65. (Oxford, London, Edinburgh: Blackwell Scientific Publications)

111. Dickerson, J.W.T. (1981). Nutrition, brain growth and development. In Connolly, K.J. and Prechtl, I.H.F.R. (eds.) *Maturation and Development – Biological and Psychological Perspectives*, pp. 110–30. (London: William Heinemann)

112. Hess, H.H., Bass, N.H., Thalheimer, C. and Deverakonda, R. (1976). Gangliosides and the architecture of human frontal and rat somatosensory isocortex. *J. Neurochemistry*, **26**, 1115–21

113. Dickerson, J.W.T., Merat, A. and Yusuf, H.K.M. (1982). Effects of malnutrition on brain growth and development. In Dickerson, J.W.T. and McGurk, H. (eds.) *Brain and Behavioural Development*, pp. 73–108. (Glasgow, London: Surrey University Press (Blackie))

114. Morgan, B.L.G. and Winick, M. (1980). Effects of environmental stimulation on brain N-acetylneuraminic acid content and behaviour. *J. Nutr.*, **110**, 425–32

115. Wurtman, R.J. and Fernstrom, J.D. (1975). Control of brain monoamine synthesis by diet and plasma amino acids. *Am. J. Clin. Nutr.*, **28**, 638–47

116. Dickerson, J.W.T. (1988). Nutrition and disorders of the nervous system. In Dickerson, J.W.T. and Lee, H. (eds.) *Nutrition in the Clinical Management of Disease*, 2nd edn., pp. 326–49. (London, Baltimore, Auckland: Edward Arnold)

117. Fraser, W.I. and Minns, R.A. (1992). Mental handicap. In Campbell, A.G.M. and McIntosh, N. (eds.) *Forfar and Arneil's Textbook of Paediatrics*, 4th edn., pp. 713–918. (Edinburgh: Churchill Livingstone)

118. Shonkoff, J.P. (1992). Mental retardation. In Behrman, R.E., Kliegman, R.M., Nelson, W.E. and Vaughan, V.C. (eds.) *Nelson Textbook of Pediatrics*, 14th edn., pp. 94–8. (Philadelphia, Sydney, Tokyo: W.B. Saunders Co., Harcourt Brace Jovanovich, Inc.)

119. Barnes, N.D. (1992). Metabolic and endocrine disorders: Part II – Endocrine disorders. In Robertson, N.R.C. (ed.) *Textbook of Neonatology*, 2nd edn., pp. 799–821. (Melbourne, New York, Tokyo: Churchill Livingstone)

120. Wraith, E. (1994). Inborn errors of metabolism. *Med. Int.*, **22**, 1, 34–8

121. Rezvani, I. and Auerbach, V.H. (1992). Defects in metabolism of amino acids: Tryptophan. In Behrman, R.E., Kliegman, R.M., Nelson, W.E. and Vaughan, V.C. (eds.) *Nelson Textbook of Pediatrics*, 14th edn., pp. 315–16. (Philadelphia, London, Tokyo: W.B. Saunders Co., Harcourt Brace Jovanovich, Inc.)

122. Rezvani, I. and Auerbach, V.H. (1992). Defects in metabolism of amino acids: Methionine. In Behrman, R.E., Kliegman, R.M., Nelson, W.E. and Vaughan, V.C. (eds.) *Nelson Textbook of Pediatrics*, 14th edn., pp. 312–14. (Philadelphia, London, Tokyo: W.B. Saunders Co., Harcourt Brace Jovanovich, Inc.)

123. Rezvani, I. and Auerbach, V.H. (1992). Defects in metabolism of amino acids: Valine, leucine, isoleucine and related organic acidemias. In Behrman, R.E., Kliegman, R.M., Nelson, W.E. and Vaughan, V.C. (eds.) *Nelson Textbook of Pediatrics*, 14th edn., pp. 316–22. (Philadelphia, London, Tokyo: W.B. Saunders Co., Harcourt Brace Jovanovich, Inc.)

124. Haslam, R.H.A. (1992). Miscellaneous causes of neurodegenerative disorders: Kinky hair disease. In Behrman, R.E., Kliegman, R.M., Nelson, W.E. and Vaughan, V.C. (eds.) *Nelson Textbook of Pediatrics*, 14th edn., pp. 1528. (Philadelphia, London: W.B. Saunders Co., Harcourt Brace Jovanovich, Inc.)

125. Balistreri, W.F. (1992). Metabolic diseases of the liver: Wilson disease. In Behrman, R.E., Kliegman, R.M., Nelson, W.E. and Vaughan, V.C. (eds.) *Nelson Textbook of Pediatrics*, 14th edn., pp. 1015–16. (London: W.B. Saunders Co., Harcourt Brace Jovanovich, Inc.)

126. Besley, G.T.N. (1994). Lysosomal disorders. In Clayton, B.E. and Round, J.M. (eds.) *Clinical Biochemistry and the Sick Child*, pp. 173–88. (Oxford, London, Edinburgh: Blackwell Scientific Publications)

127. Morgan, B.L.G. (1982). Effects of hormonal and other factors on growth and development. In Dickerson, J.W.T. and McGurk, H. (eds.) *Brain and Behavioural Development*, pp. 109–30. (Glasgow, London: Surrey University Press (Blackie))

128. Peters, T.J. (1996). Physical complications of alcohol misuse. In Weatherall, D.J., Ledingham, J.G.G. and Warrell, D.A. (eds.) *Oxford Textbook of Medicine*, 3rd edn., pp. 4276–8. (Oxford, New York, Tokyo: Oxford University Press)

129. Gardner-Medwin, D. (1996). Developmental abnormalities of the nervous system. In Weatherall, D.J., Ledingham, J.G.G. and Warrell, D.A. (eds.) *Oxford Textbook of Medicine*, 3rd edn., pp. 4105–22. (Oxford, New York, Tokyo: Oxford University Press)

130. Fagan, E.A. (1996). Liver and gastrointestinal disease in pregnancy. In Weatherall, D.J., Ledingham, J.G.G. and Warrell, D.A. (eds.) *Oxford Textbook of Medicine*, 3rd edn., pp. 1796–803. (Oxford, New York, Tokyo: Oxford University Press)

131. Morgan, J.B. (1988). Nutrition for and during pregnancy. In Dickerson, J.W.T. and Lee, H. (eds.) *Nutrition in the Clinical Management of Disease*, 2nd edn., 1–29. (London, Baltimore, Auckland: Edward Arnold)

132. Pratt, O.E. (1982). Alcohol and the developing fetus. *Br. Med. Bull.*, **38**, 43–52

133. Rylance, G.W. (1992). Neonatal pharmacology. In Robertson, N.R.C. (ed.) *Textbook of Neonatology*, 2nd edn., pp. 1193–1211. (Melbourne, New York, Tokyo: Churchill Livingstone)

134. Hallworth, M. and Capps, N. (1993). Individual drugs. In Freedman, D.B. and Marshall, W. (eds.) *Therapeutic Drug Monitoring and Clinical Biochemistry*, pp. 29–94. (ACB Venture Publications)

135. DiGeorge, A.M. (1992). Goiter. In Behrman, R.E., Kliegman, R.M., Nelson, W.E. and Vaughan, V.C. (eds.) *Nelson Textbook of Pediatrics*, 14th edn., pp. 1423–5. (Philadelphia, Sydney, Tokyo: W.B. Saunders Co., Harcourt Brace Jovanovich, Inc.)

136. Kelnar, C.J.H. (1992). Endocrine gland disorders. In Campbell, A.G.M. and McIntosh, N. (eds.) *Forfar and Arneil's Textbook of Paediatrics*, 4th edn., pp. 1085–171. (Edinburgh, London, Tokyo: Churchill Livingstone)

137. Gill, G.N., Brace, R.A., Fauser, B.C.J.N., Hsueh, A.J.W., Liu, J.H., Myatt, L., Rebar, R.W., Resnick, R. and Thomas, M.A. (1990). The thyroid gland. In West, J.B. (ed.) *Best and Taylor's Physiological Basis of Medical Practice*, 12th edn., pp. 811–8. (London, Sydney, Tokyo: Williams and Wilkins)

138. Huang, R.T., Lin, S.J., Kuo, P. L. and Peng, C.J. (1993). Successful management of a pregnancy with maternal phenylketonuria: report of a case. *J. Formosan Med. Assoc.*, **92**: 2, 182–4

139. Peat, B. (1993). Pregnancy complicated by maternal phenylketonuria. *Austral. NZ J. Obstet. Gynaecol.*, **33**: 2, 163–5

140. Rezvani, I. and Auerbach, V.H. (1992). Defects in metabolism of amino acids: Phenylalanine. In Behrman, R.E., Kliegman, R.M., Nelson, W.E. and Vaughan, V.C. (eds.) *Nelson Textbook of Pediatrics*, 14th edn., pp. 307–10. (Philadelphia, London, Tokyo: W.B. Saunders Co., Harcourt Brace Jovanovich, Inc.)

141. Buist, N.R.M., Kennaway, N.G. and Powell, B.R. (1992). Disorders of amino acid metabolism. In Campbell, A.G.M. and McIntosh, N. (eds.) *Forfar and Arneil's Textbook of Paediatrics*, 4th edn., pp. 1173–255. (Edinburgh, London, Tokyo: Churchill Livingstone)

142. Fitzhardinge, P.M. and Steven, E.M. (1972). The small-for-date infant. I. Later growth patterns. *Pediatrics*, **49**, 671–81

143. Fitzhardinge, P.M. and Steven, E.M. (1972). The small-for-date infant. II. Neurological and intellectual sequelae. *Pediatrics*, **50**, 50–7

144. Stein, Z., Susser, M., Saenger, G. and Marolla, F. (1975). *Famine and Human Development: Dutch Hunger Winter of 1944–1945*. (New York: Oxford University Press)

145. Gruenwald, P. (1974). Pathology of the deprived fetus and its supply line. In Elliott, K. and Knight, J. (eds.) *Size at Birth. Ciba Foundation Symposium No. 27*, pp. 3–9. (Amsterdam: Associated Scientific Publishers)

146. Wallis, S.M. and Harvey, D. (1992). Fetal growth, intrauterine growth retardation and small for gestational age babies. In Robertson, N.R.C. (ed.) *Textbook of Neonatology*, 2nd edn., pp. 317–24. (Edinburgh, London, Tokyo: Churchill Livingstone)

147. Wallis, S. and Harvey, D. (1982). The consequences of being small-for-dates at birth. *Ann. Nestle*, **40**, 30–42

148. Meadows, N.J., Ruse, W., Keeling, P.W.N., Scopes, J.W. and Thompson, R.P.H. (1983). Peripheral blood leucocyte zinc depletion in babies with intrauterine growth retardation. *Arch. Dis Childh.*, **58**, 807–9

149. Meadows, N.J., Ruse, W., Smith, M.F., Day, J., Keeling, P.W.N., Scopes, J.W., Thompson, R.P.H. and Bloxam, D.L. (1981). Zinc and small babies. *Lancet*, **11**, 1135–7

150. Aynsley-Green, A. and Soltesz, G. (1992). Metabolic and endocrine disorders: Part 1 – Disorders of blood glucose homeostasis in the neonate. In Robertson, N.R.C. (ed.) *Textbook of Neonatology*, 2nd edn., pp. 777–97. (Edinburgh, London: Churchill Livingstone)

151. Walker, V. (1994). Hypoglycaemia and hyperammonaemia. In Clayton, B.E. and Round, J.M. (eds.) *Clinical Biochemistry and the Sick Child*, pp. 87–120. (Oxford, London, Edinburgh: Blackwell Scientific Publications)

152. Graham, F.K., Ernhardt, C.B., Thurston, C.B. and Craft, M. (1962). Development three years after perinatal anoxia and other potentially damaging newborn experiences. *Psychol. Monogr.*, **76**, 1

153. Dalton, R.F., Forman, M.A. and Muller, B.A. (1992). Psychosocial problems. In Behrman, R.E., Kliegman, R.M., Nelson, W.E. and Vaughan, V.C. (eds.) *Nelson Textbook of Pediatrics*, 14th edn., pp. 56–7. (Philadelphia, London, Tokyo: W.B. Saunders Co., Harcourt Brace Jovanovich, Inc.)

154. Wharton, B.A., Scott, P.H. and Turner, T.L. (1994). The newborn. In Clayton, B.E. and Round, J.M. (eds.) *Clinical Biochemistry and the Sick*

Child, pp. 25–59. (Oxford, London, Edinburgh: Blackwell Scientific Publications)

155. Beischer, N.A. and Mackay, E.V. (1986). Fetal distress: umbilical cord accidents. In *Obstetrics and the Newborn – An Illustrated Textbook*, pp. 434–42. (London, Philadelphia, Hong Kong: Baillière Tindall)

156. Beischer, N.A. and Mackay, E.V. (1986). Asphyxia and resuscitation. In *Obstetrics and the Newborn – An Illustrated Textbook*, pp. 579–85. (London, Philadelphia, Hong Kong: Baillière Tindall)

157. Wennberg, R.P. (1992). Gastroenterology: Part I – Bilirubin physiology. In Robertson, N.R.C. (ed.) *Textbook of Neonatology*, 2nd edn., pp. 605–17. (Edinburgh, London, Tokyo: Churchill Livingstone)

158. Mowat, A.P. (1992). Gastroenterology: Part I – Disorders of the liver and biliary system. In Robertson, N.R.C. (ed.) *Textbook of Neonatology*, 2nd edn., pp. 619–33. (Edinburgh, London, Tokyo: Churchill Livingstone)

159. Van Praagh, R. (1961). Diagnosis of kernicterus in the neonatal period. *Pediatrics*, **28**, 870–6

160. Simeon, D.T. and Grantham-McGregor, S.M. (1990). Nutritional deficiencies and children's behaviour and mental development. *Nutrition Res. Reviews*, **3**, 1–24

161. Idjradinata, P. and Pollitt, E. (1993). Reversal of developmental delays in iron-deficient anaemic infants treated with iron. *Lancet*, **341**, 1–4

162. Golden, M.N.H. (1988). Marasmus and kwashiorkor. In Dickerson, J.W.T. and Lee, H.A. (eds.) *Nutrition in the Clinical Management of Disease*, 2nd edn., pp. 88–109. (London: Edward Arnold)

163. Lien, N.M., Meyer, K.K. and Winick, M. (1977). Early malnutrition and 'late' adoption: a study of their effects on the development of Korean orphans adopted into American families. *Am. J. Clin. Nutr.*, **30**, 1734–9

164. Wharton, B.A. (1992). Protein energy deficiency. In Campbell, A.G.M. and McIntosh, N. (eds.) *Forfar and Arneil's Textbook of Paediatrics*, 4th edn., pp. 1257–98. (Edinburgh, London: Churchill Livingstone)

165. Chisolm, J.J. (1992). Increased lead absorption and lead poisoning. In Behrman, R.E., Kliegman, R.M., Nelson, W.E. and Vaughan, V.C. (eds.) *Nelson Textbook of Pediatrics*, 14th edn., pp. 1788–91. (Philadelphia, London, Tokyo: W.B. Saunders Co., Harcourt Brace Jovanovich, Inc.)

166. Senft, K.E. and Pueschel, S.M. (1990). Lead poisoning in childhood. In Pueschel, S.M. and Mulick, J.A. (eds.) *Prevention of Developmental Disabilities*, pp. 319–33. (Baltimore, London: Paul Brookes Publishing Co.)

167. Lin-Fu, J.S. (1970). Lead poisoning in children. In *Public Health Service Publication No 2108*. (Washington, DC: U.S. Government Printing Office)

168. Smith, H.D. (1964). Paediatric lead poisoning. *Arch. Environ. Hlth.*, **8**, 256–61

169. Hoefer, A. and Hardy, M.C. (1929). Later development of breast fed and artificially fed infants. *J. Am. Med. Assoc.*, **92**, 615–19

170. Lucas, A., Marley, R., Cole, T.J., Lister, G. and Leeson-Payne, C. (1992). Breast milk and subsequent intelligence quotient in children born preterm. *Lancet*, **339**, 261–4

171. Makrides, M., Neumann, M., Simmer, K., Pater, J. and Gibson, R. (1995). Are long-chain polyunsaturated fatty acids essential nutrients in infancy? *Lancet*, **345**, 1463–8

172. Feldman, W. and Feldman, M.E. (1996). The intelligence on infant feeding. *Lancet*, **347**, 1057

173. Gale, C.R. and Martyn, C.N. (1996). Breast feeding, dummy use, and adult intelligence. *Lancet*, **347**, 1072–5

174. Thudichum, J.L.W. (1884). Quantitative relations of the immediate principles and constituents of the brain. In *A Treatise on the Chemical Constitution of the Brain*, pp. 231–60. (London: Baillière, Tindall and Cox)

Index